TAKE CHARGE
of Your CHRONIC PAIN

The Latest Research, Cutting-Edge Tools,
and Alternative Treatments for Feeling Better

PETER ABACI, MD

life

Guilford, Connecticut
An imprint of Globe Pequot Press

Dedicated to Pamela, Anthony and Gabriella for your unconditional patience, support, and love, with all my heart.

life

GPP Life is an imprint of Globe Pequot Press.

Text design by Sheryl Kober
Layout by Kevin Mak
Cover design by Jane Sheppard
Interior photographs by Peter Abaci and Ric Iverson
Illustrations on page 94 by James Hummel
Illustrations on page 156 by David Sullivan

Library of Congress Cataloging-in-Publication Data
Abaci, Peter.
 Take charge of your chronic pain : the latest research, cutting edge tools, and alternative treatments for feeling better / Peter Abaci.
  p. cm.
 ISBN 978-0-7627-5409-0
 1. Chronic pain. I. Title.
 RB127.A225 2010
 616'.0472—dc22
                                    2009036919

Printed in the United States of America
10 9 8 7 6 5 4 3 2

Contents

Introduction

As is the case with many of my peers, my interest in becoming a pain doctor grew out of my background in anesthesiology. During my anesthesia residency at the University of Southern California, one of my teachers issued this challenge: See to it that our patients wake up after surgery without any pain. If you've ever walked through a post-anesthesia recovery room in a teaching hospital and heard all the moans and groans, you know that is not an easy task. It requires giving people enough strong, intravenous pain medication so they will feel comfortable, but not so much that they won't wake up. I got to be pretty good at that game, and by the time I became chief resident during my last year I had perfected it. And when I did my senior elective in pain medicine, I learned that there were special procedures that I could perform as an anesthesiologist that could make people feel better instantly. I couldn't think of a cooler career choice.

Shortly after graduating, I decided to open my own practice. Most of my peers looked for secure jobs with established medical groups or joined large institutions where they received a salary and a steady supply of patients. I heard over and over again from older physicians about how difficult things had become in private practice, but what the heck did I know?

I soon learned how difficult it was to start an independent practice. Fully loaded with high hopes and plenty of type A habits, I left the house at 6:00 a.m. each day to get a jump on my work. There was no time to "waste" on breakfast, so I often grabbed a cappuccino and a scone from one of the local coffee spots. By noon I would be starving and often indulged in whatever I could lay my hands on, like take-out Chinese or, better yet, hospital food. I was so busy I usually spent most of the weekend at my office dictating reports and doing other catch-up work. Family time was extremely limited, and it hurt me when my five-year-old son drew a picture of his family and I wasn't in it. But his teacher assured me that this was common

1

for kids his age. Getting in enough exercise was also tough. I usually tried to cram a whole week's worth in at once by playing basketball for a few hours on Saturday morning, running as hard as possible.

I had been a lifelong soccer player, so my knees had suffered through the usual wear and tear. Everything was all right, however, until I suffered my first anterior cruciate ligament (ACL) tear when I was in my late twenties. ACL tears are common in pivoting sports like skiing, soccer, and football. I was playing in a league of mostly immigrants who spoke little English in an economically challenged part of Los Angeles. They were great guys, but dedicated to the sport; so dedicated, in fact, that when I tore my ACL, one of my teammates, who worked at the hospital where I was training, pulled off my shorts and gave them to someone else so he could take my place (The game must go on!). My right knee was too swollen and painful to walk on, so I had to roll my body to the sidelines, in my underwear, until one of my colleagues came to help me get home. Despite the injury I hobbled through my duties as chief resident without missing any time and, with a little surgery and rehabilitation, I eventually felt pretty good.

As I reached my thirties, I noticed I was becoming less coordinated when playing sports and was adding inches around my waist. It was during one of those Saturday morning basketball games, while I was running, that my right knee seemed to explode. As I lay on the court, pounding the floor with my fist in frustration and anger, I was thinking: "What did I do to deserve this? I was just running down the court, for heaven's sake!" Then I realized what had happened. I had already torn my ACL during that soccer game years before—this time I managed to tear just about everything I possibly could in that same knee. I thought it had hurt a lot the time before, but this time it was much worse. Some of the guys helped me up (with my shorts on, this time) and I eventually drove the two miles home, using only my left foot.

Surgery repaired the damage to my knee, but the pain was intense, especially at night. I could barely sleep for the next three or four months. Medications didn't seem to help much, and the nausea and constipation weren't fun either. About a week after the surgery, I went back to a full work schedule; being self-employed, I had no choice.

Each night I went home in agony, with my entire right leg swollen even though I was wearing a compression stocking. My armpits were sore from bounding around on crutches all day, and I started to notice that I was having a real hard time remembering things. People would tell me something, and fifteen minutes later I would struggle to recall what they had said. Experiencing that forgetfulness reminded me that many of my patients had told me, fearfully, that their minds did not seem to work nearly as well as they once did when their pain problems started. Although I was always at a loss to explain this phenomenon, I had consoled them with the news that they were not alone in their complaints. Now I was joining the ranks of the forgetful.

I was flat-out depressed. Many of my patients had told me they, too, became depressed once their pain had settled in. They described it as "feeling hopeless," "feeling helpless," "having a lot of dark thoughts," and "questioning the worth of living."

Getting from place to place was a struggle; I felt trapped in my body. Climbing up and down the stairs in my home exacerbated my pain. It was an ordeal! Even simply watching the nightly news, listening to the parade of terrible events and dire predictions, seemed to make my knee hurt more. I could feel the bad news go from the newscasters' lips right into my knee.

Yet little had changed. My wife still loved me, my kids were still adorable, and my job was still clicking. The only difference was a knee injury. Yes, it was severe, but millions of people had recovered from similar injuries. Still, I felt like my entire life was unraveling. I'd been hearing stories like this from my chronic pain patients for years, stories of how a single injury destroyed their lives. I had always sympathized, but felt it couldn't happen to me. Now it *was* happening to me.

It was as if I was looking in the mirror and seeing not the "healthy" me but someone who very much resembled the unfortunate people my patients had been telling me about. I asked myself the same questions they had asked me so many times: Why had I not made a full recovery? Why did a physical injury make me feel so miserable inside? What did my future look like? As a doctor I always try to lend an empathetic ear and really understand what my patients are going through, but this was a lot more than I had ever bargained for. I hadn't planned on learning how to be a good doctor by being a patient and having all these problems dumped on my head!

The rest of my body wasn't faring too well, either. My weight had edged higher thanks to the inactivity; my total cholesterol had skyrocketed to 250-plus. My LDL ("bad cholesterol") was way too high, while my HDL ("good cholesterol") was way too low. When a nutritionist told me I might be developing metabolic syndrome— a precursor to diabetes and coronary artery disease—I thought "Lovely, just lovely. Not only am I hobbling around and feeling like crap, but now the crystal ball in the nutritionist's office has me getting my first heart attack at age fifty!"

I knew I had to make some major changes, so I did. They didn't happen overnight like in the movies. It was more of an evolution over time, with lots of input from a variety of sources.

A few months after my surgery, when it was still very painful for me to do much of anything, my wife suggested that I look into Pilates. "Pee-what?" I thought. Feeling desperate, I decided to give it a go. The next thing I knew, I was working with funky equipment made of springs and bars. I was amazed to discover how my injury had affected not just my right leg but my entire body, including my stomach muscles. My instructor taught me the Pilates way to breathe, and before I knew it, my body was starting to move again. Finally! And I learned slow, steady ways to get those tight, painful spasming muscles to work again. I was gradually getting stronger and more flexible. In addition to discovering how an injury to one body part affects the whole body and being introduced to new ways of breathing, I learned exercises that helped me work through those affected areas when I was stuck, when I didn't know what to do.

I didn't lose any weight during the first post-injury year, but I didn't give up. During the first year, I began to learn about things I hadn't been taught in medical school, things like inherited body type, antioxidants, and the glycemic index. I substituted green tea for my morning dose of cappuccino and took time to prepare healthy breakfasts and lunches. I still left the house at 6:00 a.m. every day, but I went to the gym first and then to work. Because I was unable to run, I started cycling to get some aerobic exercise and enjoy the outdoors. I also stopped spending weekends at the office, devoting the time to my family instead. After about three years of consciously managing my health, I was back down to my high school body weight.

I was becoming increasingly intrigued by some of the Eastern practices, such as yoga. Too chicken to walk into a yoga studio and dive into a class, I jumped when I came across an opportunity to take some private lessons from an instructor. The physical postures were very helpful, but what I learned about myself was amazing. For example, I discovered there was a very tight area in the middle of my back that kept me from assuming certain positions. I learned that the spot seemed to be filled with sadness and other intense emotions that seeped out when I did back bends or other exercises that took a lot of energy. Opening up about my emotions was never a strength of mine. Reliving negative experiences only seemed to make me feel worse, so I tended to avoid doing that. But I came to realize that I "hid" negative energy in parts of my body and later channeled it into injured parts, like my knee, when under stress.

Both yoga and Pilates taught me about *fear*. I'm really uncomfortable with being upside down; I like the control I have when my feet are on the ground. Fortunately, one of my yoga instructors was hell-bent on teaching me how to do headstands and handstands despite the angst I felt about doing so, which was clearly reflected in my body language. It took me many months to get to the point where I could do a handstand next to a wall, but all that work—and failure—taught me a lot about balance and movement and how to work through fear without giving up.

Along the way I learned other valuable lessons about how to live with balance and harmony among family, work, and self. One summer I discovered a charming resort and fishing town along the Mediterranean, which has since become a refuge for my family and me. My time there is really very simple. I watch the people, take photographs, and chat with the local shop owners. I walk a lot, mostly up and down hills. My lunches with my family are slow and can last for hours. I've found that if I eat slowly, walk often and far, breathe fresh air, and smile at others, my batteries can be recharged in a week or less.

I bet you're thinking that with yoga and Pilates, a good diet and exercise, and lots of time and fun with my family, my knee must be as good as new and my life rosier than ever. Well, guess again. I still have chronic pain, and my knee crackles like ground glass every time I bend it. There was no magical cure, but I learned how to take care of my knee so that I can limit my discomfort while leading a very active life. As a whole I'm much healthier now, physically and mentally, than I have been at any point in my life, and it has helped me become a wiser and more effective physician. For all that I am grateful.

The story I have to tell is not about quick fixes and short-term gains, but how you can reach your greatest potential and maintain it for the rest of your life. What this book has to offer comes not only from my expertise as a pain doctor, but also from the goals we have in common and the oneness in spirit we share.

In this book I'll tell you what I've learned from my patients about overcoming chronic pain, my own experience, and the latest research. I will introduce you to the greatest tools I know that will allow you to take charge—and stay in charge—of you. The alternative, unfortunately, is to continue to let pain manage you, which I imagine is no longer acceptable if you are taking time to read this book. These tools are designed to help you address the very core of what stands in your way of forward progress. That includes basic but often overlooked items, such as what exercises to do and which foods to eat, as well as deeper pursuits, like practicing proper meditative breathing, using your brain to heal instead of harm, and improving relationships through proper communication techniques. You will learn the importance of a variety of concepts, including acceptance, the fear of reinjury, the pain matrix, balanced living, and the role of modern medicine. Lesson after lesson will demonstrate how managing chronic pain is directly linked to your total health and well-being.

Some parts of understanding and treating chronic pain are understood, and others are not. The problem is that too few people understand, and too many misunderstand. Part I of this book, "Truth," will help you understand the difference, because if you don't, there is a good chance that the medical system you rely on won't either, and you will find your condition gets worse, not better. Part II, "Think," introduces key topics everyone with chronic pain should understand, including stress, how the brain deals with pain, inactivity, and the mind/body/spirit connection. Part III, "Dare," introduces the Seven Steps to an Extreme Makeover and delves into the many empowering things you can do to manage your pain and thrive.

I wish I was an alchemist with a magic potion that would make your pain melt away. Instead I offer you wisdom and guidance to accompany you on your journey.

Live well, stay balanced, and infect others with good humor!

PART I:
TRUTH

CHAPTER 1

Introducing Good Health

When I walked into the exam room to meet Esther for the first time, she was sitting on the floor with her frail frame tucked in a fetal position. She initially avoided making eye contact, perhaps embarrassed to be meeting with a strange doctor for the first time in such a state. Disheveled and tearful, she just shook her head when asked questions. A thirty-something former alcoholic, Esther was single, socially isolated, and overwhelmed by her pain despite taking large dosages of powerful pain medications like Oxycontin. She had seriously considered suicide as a way out.

Today Esther is an attractive and successful professional who smiles brightly, dates, exercises regularly—and takes no medications. She still has pain, but she feels she is *in control.* Her transformation begs the question: How can one person exist at two opposite poles of the human spectrum *while living with the same exact health problems*? How does someone with pain in the neck, arms, and lower back go from curling up into a ball to hide from the world to becoming vibrant and engaged in a matter of mere months?

The answer is twofold. The first part is obvious, which is that Esther finally received the right treatment for her condition. This answer satisfies our basic assumption that modern medicine has the right pill or surgery for whatever ails us. Most of us go to the doctor with the expectation that whatever is bothering us can be explained by a well-defined disease mechanism, and that we will be given a specific, effective remedy that will make things much better in a short amount of time.

The second part of the answer is less obvious: Esther needed to get rid of treatments and opinions she did not need. This is a necessary part of the healing process. Think about cooking. Even if you put the right combination of tomatoes, garlic, olive oil, and basil into your famous pasta sauce, it just won't taste right if you also toss in several random ingredients. All it takes is one wrong flavor to ruin the whole dish. When we feel really rotten, we can easily lose our perspective and become more likely to go out and try something—anything—with the hope that it will help. Unfortunately, that approach can set us way back by leading us in misguided directions. Positive change can't occur when negative factors continue to hold things up.

A Deeper Understanding of Pain

Standard medical treatments can certainly help when you are in pain, but if you are not careful, they can also stand in the way of progress. Esther showed up at my center with a trail of failed treatments, prescriptions, surgeries, and above all, attitudes about chronic pain behind her; all contributed in some way to her near-complete collapse. I am convinced that she is just one of millions who is unwittingly given care with deleterious effects.

Unfortunately, there are no simple recipes to ease common chronic pain problems like low back pain or fibromyalgia. I was never given a book of tables or flow charts in medical school that laid out exactly what to do and what not to do when faced with a patient with chronic pain. I received my formal training in pain management at the highly regarded University of California, San Francisco, where I was exposed to some of the most accomplished and respected leaders in my field. I came to appreciate how complex and all encompassing chronic pain truly is, but I left with no blueprint describing how to resurrect the Esthers I would soon meet.

Acute Pain and Chronic Pain

It's important to understand the difference between chronic and acute pain. Acute pain is what you experience when you first get injured. It is caused by tissue damage and the swelling and inflammation that come along with it. Once the injury starts to heal, the inflammation subsides and the acute pain starts to resolve. This type of discomfort serves to protect you from further damage. For example, if you sprain an ankle, it becomes acutely swollen and too painful to walk on. When it hurts that much, you instinctively avoid placing weight on it, because using the ankle at that point would only make it more inflamed and interrupt the natural healing process. The acute pain goes away when the sprain resolves, allowing you to walk safely once again.

Chronic pain, on the other hand, is pain that continues after you have recovered from an acute injury. If a broken wrist has had time to heal but continues to hurt, the pain is considered chronic. As a general rule, once pain has persisted for more than six months, it meets the criteria of being considered chronic. Whereas acute pain is a *symptom* of another injury or disease, chronic pain is an *experience* that becomes its own medical problem. It can transcend the purely physical cause that set it in motion and turn into a crisis that envelopes the entire person—mind, body, and spirit.

As you will soon see, chronic pain can touch everything in your life, including how you feel, sleep, move, and relate to others. Once pain becomes chronic, it no longer protects you from further injury. In fact, it can do just the opposite: Chronic pain can shut you off from doing the things you need to do to heal. All of a sudden, *not* using something that has healed, like a sprained ankle, actually makes the ankle hurt more and grow weaker. Unlike acute medical problems, chronic pain problems are not easily cured with surgeries or antibiotics. Relying purely on such physical treatments leaves many important parts of the puzzle untouched.

It's a Widespread Problem

The "chronic pain stakes" are high; my guess is they are much higher than you realize. Chronic pain is estimated to affect one in six Americans—or some fifty million out of a total population of three hundred million—and has become the third leading cause of impairment, accounting for one hundred billion dollars in lost productivity and health costs annually. There is a good chance that chronic pain will affect every family, so we should all take notice.

The "chronic pain stats" are fairly well-known, but few people realize how much of a health risk chronic pain has become. When the lives of millions of people are disrupted, the fallout is alarming. For example, the reduction in physical activity that often accompanies chronic pain inevitably leads to weight gain—sometimes tremendous amounts. Once obesity sets in, there is an increased risk of developing a myriad of undesirable medical problems, including diabetes, arthritis, coronary artery disease, and stroke. And chronic pain often triggers ongoing stress—a silent killer that sets the stage for chronic diseases and other problems like heart attack, muscle tension, and Alzheimer's disease.

Chronic pain can destroy your emotional and social well-being. Depression is commonly associated with chronic pain, as are intense emotions like anger, grief, and fear. Such strong mood changes can easily decrease your performance at work and disrupt the harmony of your family life. This can quickly progress to an unfortunate state of social isolation, as your world grows ever smaller and smaller.

Both in numbers and fallout, chronic pain is one of the major disabling conditions of our time. And to the extent that it sets the stage for fatal diseases such as heart attacks and strokes, it is also a killer.

A Complete Education for a Complex Problem

My journey into private practice started back in 1996. Since then I have monitored firsthand virtually all the medications, procedures, and surgeries used to treat pain. At every turn I have seen lives devastated and families shattered, people unable to get out of bed and people too sad to smile. The great arsenal of modern medicine has lacked the firepower to "destroy" chronic pain. It became clear to me that we needed a new idea, a new approach, a change. But what change? What did chronic pain patients really need?

What do you do when you are faced with a perplexing challenge, but have no instructions to guide you? If you happen to think the way I do, you build something and hope to figure things out along the way. You may remember the scene from the famous Frank Capra movie *It's a Wonderful Life*, where George Bailey (played by Jimmy Stewart) holds his hands up high and proclaims, "I'm gonna build things!" I think my practice partner and I shared the same blind exuberance about wanting to improve the lives of those in pain. And so we built our own little skyscraper of a clinic, which we named the Bay Area Pain and Wellness Center. Starting from scratch we designed a special office suite that included classrooms for lectures, a gym for exercise, a quiet room for meditation, an art room for creative expression, and the more traditional exam rooms for treating patients. We created an interdisciplinary team of doctors, nurses, psychologists, physical therapists, counselors, art therapists, life coaches, Eastern Medicine practitioners, vocational experts, and exercise trainers. This team now works together to change lives, sometimes in dramatic ways.

If you think we keep our patients busy, you're right. Why? Because we try to treat the whole person, not just an arm or a leg. This means we want them to tackle many different subjects at once. Think back to when you were in school. You covered several subjects every day, from math to history to English. You wouldn't expect to be a proficient student if you were only taught one subject. Exposure to many disciplines made you a much more capable student.

I want to create highly successful students who understand the nature of chronic pain and the complex plan for controlling it, so I offer my patients a well-rounded education—not just a one-dimensional treatment—that helps them go through the simultaneous physical, emotional, and spiritual transformations necessary to conquer their pain. In order to achieve optimum health and well-being, they may have to master the "regular" subjects such as medications, meditation, and exercise, as well as less standard ones, including healthful attitudes, social connectivity, and financial independence.

Young and Healthy through Old Age

James Fries, M.D., a professor of medicine at Stanford, developed the *Theory of Compressed Morbidity. Morbidity* refers to the incidence of ill health. *Compressed morbidity* means being healthy and highly functional for most of one's lifetime, then squeezing sickness into a condensed time frame at the very end of life. In other words, disease does not occur until the end of life, at which point it would be time to die.

I realize this sounds like a geriatric fairy tale, as in "They lived healthfully ever after." But it's worth noting that Fries's recommendations for achieving compressed morbidity boil down to a few simple lifestyle habits: maintain a normal body weight, exercise regularly and vigorously, and avoid smoking. I bring this up because, of the thousands of chronic pain patients I have seen over the years, most are above their ideal body weight, have a fear of exercise, have some form of medication dependency, and, to a lesser degree, smoke. (For those who do smoke, the stress of dealing with pain seems to increase the urge to light up.)

My goal in writing this book is to help you feel young and healthy throughout your long and productive life. Doing so means shedding your dependence on doctors like me, feeling better while needing less medication, developing an active and strong body, breaking free of the mental and emotional traps created by dysfunctional thinking, and a whole lot more. The early chapters of this book look at the world of pain management that has largely been hidden from the public's view. Expect full disclosure. The middle part will help you better understand your most valuable ally in taking charge of your pain: you. The third part will introduce you to what I have found to be the most essential skills and tools for managing pain and taking charge of your life.

As you progress through the pages of this book, remember the powerful lesson I learned from Esther: *She only stopped being sick when she ceased acting like a patient.* When she was being a patient and taking the potent painkillers she had been prescribed, she continued to experience terrible pain and could barely move her body. Even though she tried a variety of strong antidepressants and anti-anxiety medicines, she remained horribly depressed and feared for her future. Staying in the house except when she had to go to doctor appointments may have seemed necessary at the time, but that didn't make her any better, either.

It wasn't until she left the patient role behind and made dramatic lifestyle changes—including exercising daily, giving up addictive painkillers, opening up lines of communication, and changing the way she viewed herself—that things finally started improving for her. In other words, *when she adopted the behaviors of the healthy, she became well.* All of her problems didn't magically disappear; they instead became a whole lot easier for her to manage.

Doctors and scientists already know that our most common chronic diseases, like diabetes, heart disease, and arthritis, are intimately linked to lifestyle factors, including nutrition, exercise, smoking, and stress. Esther taught me that the most powerful treatment to fight chronic pain is not the strongest drug or latest surgery, but rather the immersion of the self into habits designed to boost total wellness—mind, body, and spirit. I'm here to teach you the best ways I know of to do that for life.

Are You Suffering?

Here is a quick quiz I created to help you understand yourself better. It won't give you a "number" to tell you how much you hurt—because only you know that—but it can help you identify problem areas and figure out which questions you should raise with your doctors, chiropractors, physical therapists, and other health care providers so they can better serve your needs. I suggest you repeat this test in six to twelve months and compare those results with today's to get a sense of what has changed in your life.

Circle the answer (A, B, C, or D) that best describes you or your situation:

1) Over what proportion of the day do you experience pain?
   a. Rarely.
   b. 25 percent.
   c. 50 percent.
   d. Most of the day.

2) How well can you perform self-care activities like grooming and dressing?
   a. I can perform them without help.
   b. I can perform them if I go very slowly and take breaks.
   c. I need help with a few self-care tasks.
   d. I need help with the majority of my self-care activities.

3) Which describes your walking tolerance?
   a. I can walk over a mile.
   b. I am limited to a few blocks.
   c. I depend on assistive devices like canes and walkers.
   d. Zero; I need a wheelchair.

4) How many stairs can you climb?
   a. At least two flights.
   b. One flight.
   c. A few.
   d. Zero.

5) How much leisure time do you spend on the computer each day?
   a. Less than ten minutes.
   b. Ten to twenty minutes.
   c. More than an hour.
   d. Most of the day.

6) How much time do you spend in quiet meditation or prayer?

a. At least ten minutes a day.

b. Briefly each day.

c. Maybe once a week.

d. Practically never.

7) How much total sleep do you get each night?

a. Seven hours or more.

b. Five to six hours.

c. Three to four hours.

d. Less than three hours.

8) How has pain affected your sexual activity?

a. It has not changed.

b. It has decreased by about a half.

c. It occurs about once a month.

d. It is non-existent.

9) How well do you walk?

a. My gait looks normal.

b. I have a slight limp.

c. I need assistance.

d. I'm not really walking outside of the house.

10) During a typical day, how social are you?

a. I talk to more than seven people in person or by phone.

b. I may speak to two or three people.

c. I avoid social contact as much as possible.

d. I try not to leave my house or bedroom.

11) How much do you limit your recreational activity because of chronic pain?

a. Almost never.

b. About 25 percent of the time.

c. Most of the time.

d. I no longer engage in recreational activity.

12) How often do you exercise?
   a. Almost daily.
   b. Twice a week.
   c. Once a week.
   d. Never.

13) How often do you worry that you are sicker than your doctors, family, and friends realize?
   a. Never.
   b. Once or twice a month.
   c. Weekly.
   d. Every day.

14) How does your family react to your pain?
   a. They are sympathetic to my situation.
   b. They don't let me do too much so that I don't get injured.
   c. They are unwilling to take me seriously.
   d. They avoid interacting with me.

15) How often do you engage in enjoyable activities?
   a. Most days.
   b. A few times a week.
   c. Occasionally.
   d. Practically never.

16) You believe your best years are
   a. in the present.
   b. in the future.
   c. in the past.
   d. hard to gauge.

17) Compared to your days before chronic pain set in, how would you describe your ability to remember things today?
   a. It is just as good as it was before.
   b. It is occasionally difficult to remember things.

c. It is not nearly as good as it used to be.

d. It is poor; I have a lot of trouble concentrating.

18) How do you feel about your future?

a. I am hopeful.

b. I think I may get better with help.

c. My chronic pain won't change.

d. My future looks grim.

19) How often do you think about your pain?

a. Rarely.

b. Briefly, about once a day.

c. At least a couple of times every day.

d. At least every few hours.

20) In general, how do you feel?

a. Supported by others.

b. More detached from others than before chronic pain set in.

c. Lonely.

d. Isolated and nervous about your health.

21) How often do you use caffeine to get through the day?

a. Rarely or never.

b. Usually once, in the morning.

c. Twice a day.

d. Several times a day.

22) During the past four weeks, how often have you felt tense?

a. A couple of times.

b. Several times.

c. Almost every day.

d. Just about all the time.

If you circled lots of Cs and Ds, it is fair to say that right now the quality of your life is significantly limited by your chronic pain.

You may be struggling on a day-to-day basis with functional activities such as grooming, grocery shopping, and preparing healthy meals. Cs and Ds, as opposed to As and Bs, on some of these questions also suggest that you may be struggling emotionally with how you feel about yourself and your relationships with others. Your answers may also shed some light on your perceptions of the meaning of pain in your life, now and in the future.

Consider repeating this test in the future to help you identify the areas in which you are progressing and those in which you may need more assistance and focus.

Before I teach you how to master the good habits that boost total wellness—body, mind, and spirit—and help you manage your chronic pain, I first need to help you weed out misguided ideas or treatments that stand in the way of your success. So let's spend a little time figuring out how to wipe the slate clean so we can work more effectively.

CHAPTER 2

If It Ain't Broke, Don't Fix It: Don't Let Your Doctor Treat the Wrong Problem

Over the last twelve years, I have treated literally thousands of patients with chronic pain. One of the most disturbing parts of my job is witnessing how much additional suffering and anguish many of them experience because of the medical treatments with which they have been provided. Often what I help patients with is not managing their chronic pain, but the complications and side effects of the treatments they have received to help treat the pain! I'm not talking about negligence or malpractice or even rare complications, but rather negative, unforeseen consequences of common medical interventions, such as surgeries, at the hands of well-respected and experienced doctors.

Living with and trying to manage chronic pain are challenging enough without complicating and prolonging the problem with the very medical treatments that are supposed to relieve it. Ineffective treatments and unsatisfactory results, though not intentional on anyone's part, can waste valuable years of our lives that we never get back. We may lose days at work, miss family functions, and just have fewer days spent doing things we enjoy.

By identifying common misconceptions and practices that don't address the full scope of chronic pain, I will show you how to avoid additional suffering caused by trying to "fix" something that isn't really "broken."

History Repeats Itself

In the winter of 1799, a happily retired George Washington spent several hours on his horse in a snowstorm inspecting his property. Unfortunately he became ill, developing symptoms of a sore throat and fever and a respiratory tract infection. His illness may have progressed to what we would today consider pneumonia.

Washington, our beloved first president and founding father, died within days of developing this illness. Tragically, modern historians believe it was not the illness that killed him, but the treatment he received from his doctors. Washington probably went into shock and died from his medical treatment, which included bloodletting—a popular medical treatment during the colonial period that involved covering patients in leeches. It was used to treat maladies such as pneumonia, leprosy, scurvy, and herpes. Apparently about four pounds of blood was removed from poor George, ultimately contributing to his death.

Bloodletting actually goes back to ancient times as a treatment for all kinds of symptoms and diseases. Galen, the famous Greek physician, later came up with detailed formulas to figure out how much blood to draw out of each patient, based on variables like age and the weather. So why am I turning Transylvanian on you and bringing up these bloody stories about clinicians whose ideas can now easily be classified as outdated? Well, Washington's example illustrates an entrenched medical philosophy that goes back to the beginnings of recorded history. There seems to be an unwritten force in the universe that tells doctors and patients to *do something* and that doing something is better than doing nothing, even if the consequences might make things worse.

Beware of the Quick Fix

There is an expectation in our society that modern medicine should be able to *fix* or *cure* any problem. For many medical problems there are indeed remedies that lead to resolution, so much so that we are able to quickly get back on track and move on with our lives. Today if we get pneumonia, our doctor can prescribe an antibiotic that rids the offending bacteria from our lungs in as quickly as a few days. If our blood pressure is too high, we don't fret over figuring out why we have the problem; we just get on the right antihypertensive medication to get the numbers back to normal, thereby "curing" the high blood pressure. In fact we spend a lot of time checking on those numbers, over and over, to make sure we keep them in the right range. Much less attention is given to examining what factors contributed to the hypertension in the first place and trying to correct them. Why worry about cutting out the salty french fries when the medications seem to put the blood pressure in a decent range?

Unfortunately the *cure it* or *fix it* approach doesn't work with chronic pain and problems that contribute to chronic pain. In fact, many chronic pain sufferers have learned the hard way that putting too much emphasis on fixing what they *think* is the reason for their pain can actually cause more problems and broken promises of success. Some days in my clinic I feel like I am treating people who come in covered in leeches.

Chronic pain is, in some respects, like other chronic medical problems, but our medical community does not approach it in the same way. Chronic diseases prevalent in our society, such as diabetes or hypertension, are not considered *curable,* but health care professionals still offer specific treatment options that focus more on *managing* the problem than trying to cure the disease. Diabetes sufferers are taught to implement lifestyle changes, such as checking their blood sugars and changing their diets. There are no such measures taken for managing chronic pain. It would seem silly to diagnose a patient with diabetes and then spend time trying to *cure* the condition instead of implementing measures to help control blood sugars. We know that when our blood sugar gets too high, it can be a life-threatening situation, and we also know that there isn't a simple cure to make diabetes go away.

So why, when our health care system is presented with challenging chronic pain problems, does it overemphasize finding a *fix* and underemphasize managing the numerous ailments that go along with it?

What differentiates chronic pain from diseases like diabetes and hypertension is the ways in which chronic pain affects our daily lives. If our blood pressure is a little high, it doesn't ruin our day. In fact, we wouldn't even know it was high unless we checked it. A pain problem, on the other hand, impacts how we sleep, work, move, walk, and get along with our friends and family. The third part of this book will help guide you toward a path of optimally managing these different integral parts of your pain.

The Hot Pursuit of a Diagnosis

Where I often see problems first arise for patients is in their preoccupation with finding a *diagnosis*. But isn't finding the diagnosis what doctors are supposed to do? Surely there must be some value to all those diplomas you see on the wall. Why spend all of that time in the waiting room if you aren't going to get answers? Believe me, doctors feel your frustration and the pressure to give you the information you so desperately crave. In fact, doctors may feel so obligated to give you a diagnosis that they lose sight of the big picture. Yes, they can find medical nomenclature that appropriately pairs with your symptoms, but if what they come up with doesn't take into consideration the full breadth of your own particular circumstances, the treatments they prescribe have little chance for success, and you may add weeks, months, or even years to your pain instead of eliminating it.

Problem solving a patient's signs and symptoms to reach a diagnosis is, indeed, one of the fundamental arts of medicine and what most doctors believe is an integral part of what they do every day. Doctors also know that patients expect them to give answers and solve problems. Let me explain how we all get our wires crossed and, as a result, how doctors fail to truly help their patients.

There is a big difference between getting a diagnosis and learning the *cause* of a problem. A *diagnosis* is a conclusion based on analysis of the problem. This implies that the diagnosis also explains what is actually causing the problem. Unfortunately, my experience has taught me to not automatically make that assumption. Having a diagnosis doesn't necessarily mean you know what is wrong with the patient or how he or she got to this point. The central problem is the pain, yes, but the patient may also be experiencing physical, emotional, psychological, lifestyle, and prescription drug–related problems. Just settling for a *diagnosis* may tell you relatively little about what you need to know to help your patient to get better.

For example, degenerative disk disease is a diagnosis. It means that the cartilage and fluid between certain vertebrae in the spine have deteriorated. A common treatment for this painful disease when it occurs in the neck is a surgery called cervical fusion. In a typical cervical fusion surgery, a surgeon fuses vertebra together with bone grafts or metal hardware to prevent motion and stabilize the area. The surgeon picks the spot or spots to fuse based on his or her assessment of where he or she thinks the trouble is coming from.

The problem is that the degenerated disk may only be a small component of the neck pain, or possibly not a factor at all. Certainly degenerated cartilage can be found with simple imaging tests, and doctors can quickly find out where the anatomical change has taken place. Therefore the diagnosis would not be, by any means, a misnomer or an inaccurate pickup by the health care team. However, the discovery may not adequately explain *why* the pain is present. Focusing all treatments and energies toward a problem that isn't really *the* problem can't be expected to yield fulfilling results—such as alleviating the neck pain.

Visualize a patient who has just been diagnosed with degenerative disk disease in the neck, also known as the cervical part of the spine. She is about forty-five and works as an administrative assistant. She spends hours keyboarding at a computer, and her boss can often come across as rude and ungrateful. If we watch our friend at work, we see that her keyboard is too high and she scrunches her shoulders when working. We also notice that every time her boss walks by, she tenses her shoulders even more. On stressful days she might have four or five cups of coffee to help her get her work done. Her commute home includes thirty minutes of driving in thick freeway traffic. Her neck seems to hurt more by the end of the day, and it feels like it is getting progressively worse. Eventually it gets so stiff that she isn't comfortable turning her head to change lanes.

Once she gets home, she has to hurry to find something to throw together for dinner for her husband and teenage son. After dinner she tries to unwind a little by reading her friends' e-mails, browsing the Web, and watching a little late-night television, especially since she doesn't sleep too well. Her husband has become increasingly frustrated and disheartened by his wife's neck pain. She doesn't seem like herself anymore, so he pressures her to see a doctor and get something done to take care of the problem.

She visits her family doctor; her husband goes too, because he is concerned and wants to make sure the doctor understands how bad things have become. Her doctor checks her out and runs some tests. The X-rays and MRI both show degenerating disks in her neck. Once she gets the reports, she and her husband agree that something needs to be done to *fix t*he problem, because she can't go on like this.

Once our friend has locked into the notion that her pain is due to degenerative disk disease, it may be difficult for her to agree to try any treatments or advice that don't directly address that problem. At this point, making needed lifestyle changes may seem too late to her. Let's say her workstation gets an ergonomic makeover, and she tries a little physical therapy. Her therapist tells her that there seems to be a lot of tension in the muscles around her neck and shoulders. "Well, of course there is," she thinks. "I have degenerative disk disease!"

She goes back to her doctor with the bad news: "My neck still hurts." If you remember, in our world the doctor *has to do something.* At this point he prescribes pain medications and refers her to an orthopedic spine specialist who treats degenerative disk disease of the neck.

The orthopedic surgeon's office looks impressive. He shows her, in detail, the films of her degenerative disk disease and where the problems lie. They discuss what surgery would look like for her, and, as he seems like a smart doctor who knows what he is doing, they set a date.

Now, let's fast-forward a year or so, when we see that our friend is now coming to see me for the first time for "pain management." She has had a two-level cervical fusion surgery. She is still in a lot of pain and has been taking strong painkillers around the clock since the surgery. She never made it back to work after the surgery, and she still can't sleep well. Now she is also feeling depressed, so her primary care doctor has prescribed an antidepressant. She spends a lot of time at home watching television, avoids her friends, and struggles just to get basic chores done each day. Her relationship with her husband has become strained. She finds herself short-tempered with him, and he feels uptight about their finances, especially since his wife is not working.

Her doctors have sent her to me *to do something*. Is there an injection I can give her that will help? Can I prescribe stronger medications to dull the pain? Her surgeon is looking at doing more tests to look for the problem and is considering more surgery if necessary.

Time out! What went wrong here? Why would a nice, hard-working woman end up like this after getting state-of-the-art tests to figure out what was wrong and treatments from highly trained and fully competent doctors and physical therapists? How many other lives start down a similar road?

A Doctor Is Not a Mechanic

It begins with how our society views health and illness. We seem to see ourselves as machines: If a part is broken, we fix it or get a new one. If a fuel pump breaks and we replace it, our car should run like new. Find the problem, treat it, and move on. Sadly, chronic pain problems don't follow this recipe, nor do human beings come with an easy-to-read owner's manual. Setting ourselves up to fail by taking this approach to chronic pain can lead to tragic consequences like broken marriages and chemical dependency. The financial effects of lost wages can be devastating to families. The emotional wear and tear on the person at the center of it all can't be measured or put into words.

Let us assume that in the hypothetical case discussed above, the X-rays of the patient's neck backed up the diagnosis of cervical degenerative disk disease. Sadly this particular diagnosis, though not inaccurate, did not help our friend get the help she needed to address her neck pain. Her preoccupation with her diagnosis may have blinded her and her providers to other important factors. For example, how bad was her workstation and how long had it been that way? Did this cause muscular imbalances in her upper body that could have been treated? What about the effects poorly managed stress from work, home, and commuting had on her pain? How about the lack of balance among work, family, and self in her life? She really wasn't spending any time on herself to manage her health. How long had it been since she had exercised or gotten any fresh air? When was the last time she did a hobby or read a great novel? When did she last hold hands with her husband?

Pain Generators

Sometimes when doctors are struggling to find a diagnosis, they look for something called a *pain generator* to help them. Be careful to not put too much trust in this concept, or you may find yourself, again, trying to fix something that isn't all that broken.

A pain generator is a structural or anatomical problem that causes pain. For example, a protruding disk in the lower back may be pinching one of the nerve roots as it travels out of the spinal canal. This might lead to sensations of pain shooting down a leg, sometimes referred to as sciatica. In this case the pain generator would be that particular disk that is pressing up against the nerve root.

For many acute problems, finding the pain generator can help your clinical team understand what is going on and provide you with appropriate care. If you have a one-month history of acute sciatica, there is a good chance that modern medicine can locate a discrete anatomical explanation for why. The problem is when this concept is carried over to chronic pain problems. Continuing to look for a purely anatomical source of your pain symptoms once they have become chronic will set you up to rely on a *diagnosis* that won't adequately describe the world you are living in. Locating a structural change that has taken place in your body and trying to *fix* it won't improve your mood, sleep, relationships, or sex life—or even stop your pain. In other words, you won't accomplish your wellness goals.

Now visualize a person with a more long-term case of sciatica caused by a pinched nerve. Let's say the sciatica has continued for twelve months. Now we see lots of changes in the muscles in the patient's back. Some are tight and stiff. She can no longer touch her toes. She has become deconditioned, because she hasn't been walking or exercising like she used to. Climbing stairs hasn't been a reality for several months. After dealing with this for a whole year, she feels sleep-deprived almost every day and easily gets irritable. Once the message of "pain" is sent from a nerve somewhere in the body to the brain, and that pain becomes chronic, that message infiltrates all the other parts of our brains and can stay there. So, taking the stress off of a pinched nerve in her lower back by removing the piece of disk that is pressing on it won't automatically undo all of these complex nerve changes in her brain, nor will it magically reverse all the physical changes her body has made. (Read more about how the brain adapts to stress and changes in thinking in chapter 7.) Learning how to retrain our brains to retrain our bodies is hard for anyone, but you will get better at it after finishing this book.

There Are No Tests to Adequately Measure Pain

Let me give you a real-life example of what can happen when there is a preoccupation with pain generators. I first met Tina under less than ideal circumstances. She was in her late thirties and had just undergone surgery—a multilevel lumbar fusion, which means she had rods and screws placed in her lower back to stabilize her spine. Her spine surgeon couldn't manage her pain while she was still in the hospital recovering from the surgery, so he asked me to help. When I approached her bedside, her eyes held a look of sheer terror. Tina couldn't verbalize to me how she felt or what had happened.

I quickly learned from her chart that she had been working in a factory when she slipped and fell on a wet floor. This fall caused her to have back pain. She was *diagnosed* with bulging disks in her back and had had one surgery on her back before this one. I also discovered that prior to her second surgery she had been taking a whopping 600 milligrams (mg) of morphine every day to help manage the pain resulting from her first surgery. This dosage is enough to sedate an elephant for a week. Her tolerance for pain medication had become so high, it was just too difficult to manage her postoperative pain after her extensive second surgery.

Undoubtedly her doctors had thoroughly investigated for pain generators to make sure this second surgery would be a complete success. Her surgeon probably meticulously measured the shape and contour of each vertebra in her spine on several different X-rays. He probably compared old MRIs to new MRIs and confirmed what disks to fuse with discography.

Discography. Never heard of it? It is a special test in which a physician places a number of eight-inch-long needles inside the disks in the lower back under X-ray visualization. "Positive disks" are painful when contrast dye is injected through the needles with pressure. It doesn't sound fun because it isn't! If the tests show a positive disk, there is a good chance a surgeon will want to fuse that level of the spine as part of a surgical procedure on the spine. The theory behind this is that when the outer collagen of the disks is torn, it can leak a jelly-like material that is usually housed inside the disks, which leads to discomfort in the back. This is known as an *annular tear.* Implanting rods and screws into the vertebra above and below the disk with the annular tear is supposed to hold it in place, which is precisely what Tina's doctors told her she needed to eliminate her low back pain.

There is some controversy in medicine over whether or not discography is a valid and useful test. Some surgeons truly believe it is a useful diagnostic tool that improves surgical outcomes. It should be pointed out that discography is a somewhat subjective test, as it relies on patient responses to pain while under considerable sedation. Relying heavily on this type of test to develop a treatment plan for chronic back or neck pain will set up many patients to fail. Tina's case proved to be an example of how looking at only one part of the problem—in this case the pain generator—is not an effective way to treat pain.

Tina didn't really recover from that second surgery. In fact, I was forced to increase her morphine to 900 mg a day to help her manage the increased level of pain. She continued to smoke cigarettes, even though research shows that tobacco can inhibit healing after back surgery. To help Tina participate better in physical therapy, her surgeon asked me to place an implantable spinal pump so that we could infuse pain medication right into her spine This didn't really help, either.

Over the next five years, Tina went on to have many more surgeries on her back. Her surgeon extended her fusion way up into her thoracic spine, the area behind the chest. This was to correct the curvature that had taken place in her spine after the first two surgeries. She was no longer able to stand up straight; instead, she had to walk bent forward over a walker. Before each surgery she received a comprehensive tutorial from her spine surgeon about the structural problems in her spine and what surgical corrections were needed to *fix* it. She remained hopeful that things were going to work out, but her situation only deteriorated.

Possibly due to her inactivity, Tina gained a lot of weight and started taking diet pills, some of which were later taken off the market by the FDA because of serious side effects. She became depressed and spent several years working with psychologists and psychiatrists.

She even entertained suicidal thoughts at one point. Her marriage of almost twenty years dissolved.

Even though I was eventually able to reduce the amount of pain medications she was taking to very small levels, the toll it took on her system was not easily reversed. Opioid medications, like morphine, can be constipating. They slow the motion of the intestines, thereby making it harder for the bowels to empty. The high dosages that Tina was exposed to for such a long time caused an almost complete shutdown of her bowels. She developed constipation to the point where she was having bowel movements about once every month. She sought help from a few different gastroenterologists, who were concerned that she might lose the use of her colon altogether and would possibly need to have the colon removed and replaced with a pouch within the next year.

I remain troubled by how a healthy young woman could go from falling on her tailbone at work to seeing her way of life deteriorate before her very eyes because the medical treatments she received caused more harm than the fall itself. I worry about how her back will hold up as she gets older after undergoing so many surgeries involving so many different levels of her spine. The odds of her ever working again under these circumstances are not good. Tina cannot make up the years that she missed her children's school functions and activities; her kids are now grown and have lives of their own. The other medical problems, like the constipation and obesity, will undoubtedly affect her health for years to come.

Through all that Tina went through, including the seeming lack of success she reaped over the years from medical treatments and surgeries, I was always surprised by her unwavering confidence in her surgeon and her willingness to go forward with whatever treatment options offered to her. She believed in the system and believed she had a right to find out what was broken and get it fixed. With each new phase she went through, she put all the blame for her pain on pain generators. Each of these structural problems carried a diagnosis with it, which became the focus of her medical attention. Tina was so hooked on getting something done to *fix her* that nothing I said ever really made her change direction. She put off or neglected many parts of her life for over eight years, waiting for someone to "get her better," and she was never open to trying to create change from within.

The Power of Words

The words we hear and believe can greatly affect the paths we choose in life. They can be liberating and life enhancing, or, as in Tina's case, they can lead to tragic consequences. Once you hear and accept a certain diagnosis, you may find yourself focusing solely on that diagnosis. Anything else that your doctors, family members, and friends have to offer concerning your pain may fall on deaf ears.

Patients often tell me surprising things they've heard from their doctors. A common statement goes something like this: "If you don't have this surgery now, you might wind up in a wheel-chair someday." I'm always shocked when a patient tells me this. Naturally, if a doctor tells you that your legs are going to stop working, you will take those words seriously. The fact that the doctor said "might" will probably fail to register, while the idea that you'll be in a wheelchair if you don't get that surgery will become a driving force behind all of your choices.

But what does this frightening proclamation really mean? It depends on whether you ask the patient or the doctor. Most patients would interpret these words to mean that paralysis is a likely result if nothing is done. The doctor, on the other hand, may have considered the chances of paralysis unlikely, but felt obligated to educate the patient by mentioning this possibility. Regardless of the doctor's intentions, many patients imagine the worst-case scenario when given threatening news.

For those who engage in *catastrophic thinking* (jumping to the worst possible interpretations of events, actions, or statements), words can be far more powerful than they were intended to be. For example, if your doctor tells you that there is degeneration of the disks in your lower back, you might immediately jump to the conclusion that you will lose the ability to walk and be bound to a wheelchair for the rest of your life. In reality your doctor said nothing like that, and the degeneration you developed might even be considered a normal part of aging. In this instance *you* have told yourself that something is more dangerous than it may be. This problem is more directly related to how the brain processes information than to the power of the words themselves.

The First Step: Ask Questions

Our health care system is geared toward doing things; doing them now and doing them aggressively. Most of the time that's a great idea. When you're having a heart attack, when a bone is broken, or an infection is raging through your body, immediate treatment narrowly focused on the problem and geared toward *fixing it now* is exactly what you need. This is especially true in obvious cause-and-effect situations, such as the blockage of a major artery in the brain that is causing a stroke or kidney failure that is causing the body to fill with toxins.

But chronic pain is a different matter. You and your doctor have to resist the temptation to fix something—anything—*now*. Rather than search only for a handy pain generator to pin all the blame on, one that will supply you with a narrowly based diagnosis, you have to take a broad view of the situation and be willing to tolerate the uncertainty of not having a diagnosis—at least, not right away, not at the expense of understanding the full implication of your pain. Finding a pain generator is great if there is one, but there is a danger of getting stuck on something that is no longer relevant.

When a new patient comes to see me, or is referred by another physician, I like to ask myself a few questions before suggesting any treatment:

- If a pain generator has already been identified, or if I locate one, is it safe to say that this is the only cause of pain? Might there be another reason—or reasons—for the pain? Once pain has become chronic, it is often multifactorial—there are many factors playing into how it turns out.
- Does the patient need validation that there is indeed physical pain? If the patient is focused on the physical cause of the pain, is he or she focusing on it so much that he or she ignores other factors? Does my diagnosis take into account any emotional or other nonphysical factors?
- Am I only looking at treatments targeting a pain generator and not taking a step back and looking to treat the whole person?
- Are there lifestyle problems contributing to the pain? Is this person overtaxed by working too hard, avoiding needed exercise, and eating the wrong foods? Does this person have outlets to relieve built-up tension?
- What problems or side effects might the patient be experiencing from medications, and how might those drugs be limiting the patient's ability to function mentally and physically?
- What if I focus on this treatment, throw all my eggs in one basket, and it doesn't help? How will the patient cope with that, having invested time, money, and hope in something that strained finances and perhaps relationships but did not bear fruit?
- When I make a recommendation for treatment, am I trying to fix something that isn't really broken? Or that really isn't the cause of the patient's chronic pain and distress? Am I being waylaid by the desire to *do something* to fix the problem, even if the "cure" threatens to make everything worse?

See Yourself as Well

Sometimes the first and most important step in dealing with chronic pain is to drop the assumption that because someone has labeled you with a diagnosis, you must be severely ill or disabled and must be "fixed" immediately by whatever means possible (which usually means powerful medicines or surgery). Get more information. Consult with several doctors, as well as physical therapists, dietitians, and other health professionals who may be able to offer you help. Don't let a few possibly misguided words trick you into seeing yourself as less capable than you really are.

For example, I sometimes see this happen with fibromyalgia, a syndrome that usually affects females and is characterized by widespread but discrete muscle pain, fatigue, insomnia, and depression. Many people begin to see themselves as disabled once they are told they have fibromyalgia—once they are labeled. Their behaviors and attitudes begin to change noticeably, and they can assume a "sick" role and retreat into a shell.

Don't let words or labels rob you of personal fulfillment. Do not disengage or sell yourself short because of a diagnosis, which may or may not be correct. Avoid the understandable temptation to put all your eggs in the pain generator basket and fixate on a diagnosis. See yourself as ready to get and stay well, rather than as *sick*. This shift alone can do a lot to help you overcome the challenges chronic pain puts before you.

You might be amazed to find out that an entire industry has grown up around the diagnosis and treatment of chronic pain. Sadly, the sicker you become and the longer you stay that way, the bigger the profits. As you will soon see, if you're not careful, you can find yourself caught in its clutches, able to do little more than hope and pray you escape unharmed.

CHAPTER 3

A Fistful of Dollars: Your Pain Is Making Someone Very Rich

"It's all about bucks, kid. The rest is conversation."
—Gordon Gekko,
from the movie *Wall Street*

Back in the 1980s, Michael Douglas brought to the big screen a vivid presentation of the intense, cutthroat competition seen in corporate Wall Street. Through his "Gordon Gekko" character, he made it clear that "greed is good" and showed what can happen when the stakes are sky high and the pressure to win unrelenting.

I bet you never thought you might be the focus of corporate takeovers, kickbacks, and large CEO bonus packages, but it turns out, you absolutely are! In fact there is a good chance that your pain is making somebody rich right now. The *chronic pain business* has become a huge multibillion-dollar industry, and the desire for ever-rising corporate profits plays a large role in guiding the care you receive.

Pen and Pad = $$$

In 2006, fifty-seven million Americans bought prescription painkillers at a cost of $13.2 billion, according to the federal Agency for Healthcare Research and Quality. This includes opioid-based pain medications, which are highly addictive and can't just be dropped cold turkey without triggering some very unpleasant withdrawal symptoms. On top of that, we spend another $2.4 billion on non-prescription painkillers and $6 billion on supplements.

People in the business of selling medications for chronic pain want their customers to continue to take them—endlessly—so the money will keep on flowing. Once someone begins taking this kind of medicine, he or she often cannot stop, which is why pain is the "gift that keeps on giving" in the eyes of the pharmaceutical industry. That's why the competition for your business is so "Gekko-like."

Let's consider how the pharmaceutical industry works: The most important step in the process of selling medications is when the doctor writes the prescription. A pen, in the doctor's hand, scribbling on a prescription pad is the Holy Grail for pharmaceutical companies. It is the key that unlocks billions of dollars in disease-treating expenses each year. If, like the pharmaceutical companies, your business depended on one simple action taking place hundreds or thousands of times each day, you would do whatever you could to see that it continued to happen.

You may be thinking that it doesn't matter what the pharmaceutical companies want; that has no influence on prescription-writing practices. After all, doctors learn which medications to use, when and how, during medical school. That is partly true. Doctors do learn the fundamentals of pharmacology in medical school. What happens after they graduate is not unlike what happens in the rest of a free-market society. It's not an exaggeration to say that medicines are "sold" to doctors just as toys are sold to children who watch Saturday morning cartoons. Today's avalanche of advertising works on both doctors and children. You can see the results in the sales figures. Simply put, doctors are victims of the same kind of advertising and salesmanship that other professionals, and consumers, are.

Throughout their careers, doctors are bombarded with marketing strategies in the form of advertisements, sales representatives, conferences, and gifts. Young physicians working in hospitals as they train as interns and residents meet attractive and articulate sales folks who sponsor meals and give them treats so they can get face time with them. Then they do their best to persuade these young doctors to use their products, rather than those of their competition. Doctors spend the rest of their careers interacting with young, polished pharmaceutical representatives whose bonuses and vacations depend on what the doctors prescribe. (Yes, doctors' prescription practices are tracked by the pharmaceutical companies, and their representatives are rewarded accordingly.) There is a reason why free pens imprinted with pharmaceutical company logos are constantly being dropped off at my office. How can I forget to prescribe a certain drug when there is a pen with its name on it in between my fingers?

If kept to a minimum, this practice could be harmless and might even help remind doctors of certain medicines or other tools. However, it is often carried to an extreme. I know of a certain physician who practically decorates his office with items donated by pharmaceutical companies. The walls of his examining rooms are covered with patient information graphs and anatomical charts, while his countertops display anatomical models and other gadgets, all stamped with the name of the generous drug companies that provided them for free. The pens in the pencil cup all bear the name of the donating pharmaceutical company, as does the paper pulled across the exam table for each new patient. In fact, the entire roll is helpfully stamped with the firm's name, lest anyone forget.

You might argue that this is just capitalism, no different from the advertisements we see all day long on television, billboards, stadium walls, buses, NASCAR drivers' uniforms and cars, and many other places. Perhaps. But what about the prescription pad this doctor has? The one that lists the appropriate medicines—in this case, antibiotics—with the company's brand-new, highly promoted antibiotic at the top of the list? In larger letters! Is that harmless advertising? When does it cross the line?

This relentless marketing pressure even appears in medical journals—almost every one of which receives corporate sponsorship through paid advertising. These journals provide a large proportion of the continuing education doctors receive once they complete their training. Reading them is a practical and common way to stay on top of new developments. I'm holding a recent copy of one of medicine's most respected and quoted journals in front of me. Studies printed in this publication are cited in major newspapers every week. When I open the cover to the first page, I see a two-page advertisement for a new antidepressant sponsored by a large pharmaceutical company, complete with a nice picture of a happy couple grocery shopping. As I look at the picture, I remember that free pens for this particular medication have already circulated through my office, as well as free croissants and coffee for my staff. This new antidepressant is actually very similar to one that came out in the 1990s, but it contains the "active ingredient" of the medication it is designed to replace. The older version is just that—old—which means its patent has run out and it is now available as a less-profitable generic pill that can be sold by other companies. Nothing has happened to "spoil" the medicine from the doctor's point of view, but from the pharmaceutical company's accountant's point of view, the pill is no good. As I flip through the pages of this journal, I see several more full-page and two-page advertisements for various medications with equally lofty qualifications.

In-person contacts with physicians and ads in scientific journals are just the beginning. The private industry sector of health care also plays a large role in continuing physician education. Doctors are required to receive continuing medical education every year to maintain their licenses, and they most often do so by attending some form of medical conference. And virtually all major medical conferences are sponsored by large, publicly traded companies, including pharmaceutical companies and medical device makers. One company can easily put tens of thousands of dollars into a single conference that may be helpful in the marketing of its product. For example, in my mail this week, I received a booklet reminding me about a large national pain management conference coming up in a few months. Not only does the booklet contain the schedule of lectures and events, but it also helpfully lists the corporate sponsors for the event. It turns out that this particular meeting, which will be in Hawaii, is sponsored by a whopping thirty-five pharmaceutical and medical supply companies, some of which are Wall Street behemoths.

All of these supporters will have exhibits in a large hall, where they can interface with doctors who attend the meeting, talk about their products, and gather e-mail addresses. Some of the larger sponsors are also offering special lunch and dinner lectures, where doctors can hear distinguished professors present a *"sermon on the mount"* about a topic in which they have expertise—which inevitably just happens to include a lot of information about the sponsoring company's products. Most of the academicians who teach doctors at these venues are also sponsored by the private industry, in addition to whatever university job they already have. In short, large medical conferences are just as important to health care companies as they are to the physicians there to learn. And they exert a lot of influence. Doctors are required to get continuing medical education every year to maintain their licenses, so they really can't avoid this process.

Winds of Change

Several years ago my state, California, adopted a new policy requiring all physicians to take continuing education classes in pain management. The idea behind it was well intentioned: to prevent the undertreatment of pain. For two decades now we've recognized that acute pain and pain associated with end-of-life care are often not adequately relieved. This new requirement was seen as a great opportunity for physicians to gain knowledge and insight into the alleviation of suffering in those with terminal illnesses and the tools for managing more complex chronic pain problems.

Unfortunately, what California doctors got was a snowstorm of lectures sponsored by large pharmaceutical companies that focused exclusively on medications and ignored all other bona fide options for treating pain. None of the other valuable pain management information like that discussed in this book was presented to California's doctors. It seemed like the only lectures that weren't about how to treat pain with medication were about *other* medications used to treat the side effects triggered by the pain medications (e.g., "If our pain medications make your patients too sleepy to do anything, you can give these other medications to keep them more awake.")

The fallout from this strong marketing—oops, I mean *educational*—push became readily apparent. When I first started practicing in the late 1990s, new patients weren't usually taking much in the way of medications for their pain. This was because their doctors weren't usually "trained" to manage medications like long-acting opioids, so they preferred to have a specialist such as myself decide what to prescribe and how to manage it.

But since doctors began taking the mandatory courses in pain management, they have become more aggressive in prescribing powerful pain pills. Over the years, I have seen a dramatic change in the amount of medicine people are already taking when they come to my office for the first time. By the time some people with complex chronic pain problems pass through my doors, they already have mile-long medication lists. Typically they have already tried at least three different types of narcotic-based medications, plus numerous adjunctive medications like sleep aids, antidepressants, muscle relaxants, antianxiety medications, and sometimes medications needed to counteract their side effects, like excessive drowsiness, nausea, and constipation. I remember seeing a patient several years ago who had a history of nodding off into his cereal bowl in the morning. Somehow I don't think snoozing in corn flakes was what the California State Medical Board had envisioned when they came up with their pain management education plan.

Instead of folks seeking my expertise on pain medications, more commonly they arrive with very long lists of medications that they have become dependent on, hoping I can clean up the mess and set their ship sailing in a different direction.

Small Steps in the Right Direction

Leaders of the medical community have recognized that gift giving—from inexpensive pens and prescription pads all the way up to lucrative consulting contracts—has gotten out of hand. For that reason several plans for restricting the gift giving have been proposed.

The Association of American Medical Colleges has suggested that medical schools and teaching hospitals adopt "policies prohibiting physicians, faculty or staff members, residents, and students from accepting any industry gifts, including industry-supplied food and meals unrelated to accredited continuing medical (CME) programs."[1] This recommendation is not binding and subject to the sort of interpretation that could keep lawyers busy for years, but it's a start. It's estimated that up to one third of medical schools have already adopted policies of this nature.

Symptom Manager, MD

Besides encouraging doctors to prescribe more pain pills, the pharmaceutical companies have indirectly yet persuasively promoted the idea that doctors can *manage* pain symptoms with even more pills.

Physicians across the country have been trained to be *symptom managers* thanks to educational grants made by the pharmaceutical industry. Many doctors have been "educated" to believe that every complaint their patients come up with should be treated with a prescription solution of some sort. If their pain is bad when they get out of bed in the morning—BAM!—provide a fast-acting narcotic medication that gets into the system immediately. If their muscles start twitching, instead of thinking about getting the muscles more conditioned to handle their workload—BOOM!—prescribe a muscle relaxant. If they are too sleepy to stay upright because of the other two medications—WHAM!—in goes a pill to boost adrenaline.

Let me share with you the story of Bridget, who had an impressive list of symptom-management pills. Bridget strained her right arm operating a cash register while working in a grocery store. She kept working for the next couple of days but had to rely on her left hand to do most of the work, which led to a strain of her left thumb.

---

1   Steinbrook, R. Physician-Industry Relations—Will Fewer Gifts Make a Difference? *NEJM* 2009; 360:6, 557–9.

Soon Bridget developed chronic pain in both of her hands and arms and was taken off work to get treatment. Her doctors tried different therapies and treatments without success. This was followed by surgeries on her left thumb and right carpal tunnel, but her pain symptoms only got worse.

During this difficult period she became extremely depressed and thought about suicide a lot. Bridget had had a hard life. Her parents divorced when she was young, and she struggled through an eating disorder as a teen and young adult. When she became older, she experienced some abusive relationships and a few divorces of her own. Once she stopped working, she lost all motivation to leave the house or interact with others.

A big focus of her medical care was on the use of medications to control her symptoms of pain, distress, and depression. Here are some of the medications that were on her list when I met her for the first time:

- Methadone
- Actiq
- Percocet
- Lexapro
- Wellbutrin
- Cymbalta
- Topamax
- Neurontin
- Provigil
- Caffeine supplements
- Mobic
- Prilosec
- Senna

Methadone, Actiq, and Percocet are opioids, or narcotic pain medications. Bridget was actually prescribed over 200 mg of methadone a day, which is a whopping dose. (Thanks to so many overdoses over the past couple of years, the FDA has put a "black box" warning on methadone—the strongest warning the agency can order a pharmaceutical company to put on its products.) Actiq contains a very potent narcotic called fentanyl. Because fentanyl has such a strong abuse potential and is so potent, Actiq is approved by the FDA only for the treatment of terminal illnesses. It is not supposed to be used for chronic pain, yet aggressive marketing by the manufacturer has persuaded many doctors to prescribe it to patients just like Bridget. Actiq typically costs thousands of dollars to take each month.

Other items on her list also concerned me. She was taking three antidepressants (Lexapro, Wellbutrin, and Cymbalta), yet she seemed horribly depressed. She was also taking two medications for "nerve pain" (Topamax and Neurontin), which, along with the opioids, impaired her cognitive functioning. She was so "prescription drugged up" that she was also prescribed two medications to keep her more alert (Provigil and caffeine). Mobic was added in the hopes of lowering her inflammation, but it also contributed to a bleeding ulcer. Because these medications have effects on the digestive system, she also needed stool softeners (Senna) and something to lower the excess acid in her stomach (Prilosec).

Despite this impressive *symptom management* list, Bridget reported debilitating pain symptoms and suicidal thoughts, and she couldn't lift or carry more than one pound of weight. Today she is off most of these medications and has received intensive treatment focused on restoring her health. As a result she is alert, more cheerful, and able to carry an eight-pound carton of milk.

Blue Pills on a Sunday Afternoon

Several years ago the multibillion-dollar pharmaceutical industry found another worthy marketing target: you! Have you noticed the steady rise in medication commercials on television? It seems as though they get bolder every year. I can't watch a professional football game on television with my son without seeing advertisements during time-outs on how to cure erectile dysfunction and become a stud muffin. Many commercials currently running focus on chronic pain–related topics such as insomnia and fibromyalgia. While I don't think it is inherently wrong for a company to advertise its products, I do believe that this incessant "marketing to the millions" gets patients to put pressure on their doctors to prescribe these particular medicines. And most of my physician colleagues agree that it is a lot easier to say yes than no to patients who ask to try—and often insist on—something they saw on television or read about on the Internet.

Expect to see more marketing directly aimed at consumers through venues like television, e-mail, text messaging, and print. In 2007 the *New York Times* reported that one manufacturer of an over-the-counter painkiller was offering an online game that would take users through blogs and social network sites as a way of targeting the under-fifty crowd.

Caught Red-Handed

It's not just the pharmaceutical companies that profit from your pain; numerous other types of health manufacturers profit too. One area of medicine that has seen rapid growth over the last two decades is spine surgery, the rate of which has risen exponentially in the United States over the last fifteen years. Spine surgery has become a commonly used treatment option for chronic back pain—one of the most prevalent forms of chronic pain in Western society—especially when other treatments have failed.

According to the National Institutes of Health, in 2000, 195 of every 100,000 people in the United States had had spine surgery. The facility fees alone for these surgeries, which is what hospitals and surgery centers charge and does not include doctor fees, was estimated to be $6.1 billion.

Then there are the fees for the hardware used in spinal fusions. Several different medical device manufacturers are involved in this industry and are, therefore, a part of the "pain business." This hardware, which includes things like plates and screws, is costly. You may wonder how expensive something like that can really be. It turns out the spinal device unit of the giant medical device manufacturer Medtronic Inc. brings in $3 billion in annual revenue!

The amount of activity by large manufacturers of implants and hardware around this burgeoning spine surgery business would make Gordon Gekko feel right at home. Let's look at what Medtronic and some of the surgeons it works with have been caught doing to generate those kinds of sales.

On July 19, 2006, the *New York Times* reported that Medtronic agreed to pay the federal government $40 million to settle a claim that the company was giving doctors kickbacks if they used its spinal implant devices. The Justice Department described what was done as "sham consulting agreements, sham royalty agreements and lavish trips to desirable locations."[2] The *Times* noted, "Complex back surgery has become a lucrative business for companies making implants, and Medtronic was accused of spending tens of millions of dollars on consulting contracts and other types of payments to prominent spine surgeons." One of the whistle-blowers described what was going on as "bribes."

Worse yet, the *Wall Street Journal* reported on September 25, 2008, that Medtronic's spinal devices unit was accused in a lawsuit of giving surgeons "a variety of incentives to use its products, including regular entertainment at a Memphis strip club, trips to Alaska and patent royalties on inventions they played no part in."[3] The *Journal* further noted that Medtronic was accused of picking up the tab for "VIP" visits to the strip club by surgeons and that the owner of this same "gentleman's club" had pleaded guilty to charges of prostitution in 2007 and closed up shop. The lawsuit alleged that Medtronic set up consulting agreements with over one hundred surgeons as a way of keeping them from using competitors' products. One surgeon was specifically cited as receiving $450,000 a year for consulting work, while another was given a helicopter ski trip in honor of his promotion at a Los Angeles hospital.

---

2   Reed Abelson. "Medtronic Will Settle Accusations on Kickbacks," *New York Times,* July 19, 2006. Accessible at www.nytimes.com/2006/07/19/business/19medtronic.html?_ r=1&pagewanted=print.

3   David Armstrong. "Lawsuit Says Medtronic Gave Doctors Array of Perks," *Wall Street Journal,* September 25, 2008.

Medtronic is not the only spinal implant device maker who has come under fire by whistle-blowers. Blackstone Medical, now owned by Orthofix International, is also under investigation for paying kickbacks for bogus consulting contracts, fake research studies, and Medicare fraud. Both companies have issued statements insisting that they have cleaned up their business practices.[4]

Am I implying that spine surgery is without merit or is a crooked branch of medicine? No, I am not. Most spine surgeons are caring, well-meaning doctors who genuinely want to help their patients and often do. However, I believe that for even well-intentioned physicians, the decision-making scales can be tipped too far in one direction by aggressive corporate business strategies, as evidenced by the billions of dollars spent on hardware. Neither am I claiming that the pharmaceutical business has no place in health care. It simply should not strangle all other forms of treatment in its wake.

Profiting from Failure

Going through a major fusion surgery is a long and arduous process for a patient. The recovery sometimes takes over a year. When the outcome is poor—for example, when it does not provide pain relief—the effects on the patient can be devastating. I have seen many suffer and be scarred by depression, medication addictions, job loss, and other problems when these surgeries don't go well.

A new diagnosis sprang up during the last two decades: failed back syndrome. This refers to patients who have had at least one spine surgery but have not improved as expected. They typically continue to experience chronic pain and some level of perceived disability. Most other countries don't perform spine surgeries at the high rate that we do in the United States. As a result, failed back syndrome does not exist in most

---

4   "Spinal Device Manufacturer Involved in Kickback Investigation." *Medical Device Link.com*, January 4, 2008. Accessible at www.devicelink.com/mddi/blog/?p=575.

of the world. Unfortunately, it is one of the biggest reasons that patients are referred to my center. It seems unfortunate that a major source of the chronic pain that I treat every day is created by the same health care system designed to alleviate it.

Even if the back surgery is successful in relieving pain, it can cause other problems. People who have had spine surgery age differently over time. The support structures of their spines seem to wear out quicker in the areas where they had the surgery, leading to advanced degeneration of the disks and joints needed to support the back. And many folks who have had one fusion surgery require at least one more back operation at some point in their lives, often because the areas above and below the fusion break down and need repair.

I can safely say that while doctors, hospitals, pharmaceutical companies, and device manufacturers will *always* profit from treating pain, it's not a sure thing for the patient.

One Question

What do the medical scientists, who prefer to act purely on the basis of evidence, think about all of this? There are differences of opinion, but a general consensus is emerging: Aggressive, *nonsurgical* rehabilitation for chronic low back pain provides long-term outcomes that are comparable to spine surgery for a lot less money. However, because there are still circumstances in which spine surgery has strong merit, there will always be a need for this surgery.

Artificial disks are now available, and this appeals to some who hope that new technology may be better than the old. I believe the jury is still out on replacing disks in people's spines and that we should not be cavalier about treatments that rely on artificial hardware to hold up our spines for years to come. For example, let's say you are fifty years old and opt to have an artificial disk put in your lower back. It is unlikely that this material will last as long as you will. So what will be the status of your spine twenty years from now? When will the disk need to be replaced? The truth is nobody really knows, and that is a chance you must be prepared to take if you undergo this surgery.

When all is said and done, I think there is one magic question you should always ask your doctor about whatever he or she recommends: *"If I was your spouse, parent, or child, is that what you want me to do?"* In other words, *"Doc, would you want your spouse to be on those medications?"* or *"Would you want your father to have that surgery?"* If your doctor's answer is *not* a resounding yes, then think seriously before you accept this advice. *I promise you there isn't anything I recommend in this book that I don't embrace as valuable to my own health or my family's health.*

I do my best to keep this perspective with my own patients. That is why some of the new discoveries about certain painkillers have me very concerned for my patients who use them. You'll see why I'm worried in the next chapter.

CHAPTER 4

Opioids: The Karl Marx of the People

Imagine you open the newspaper and read an article that says the blood pressure medicine you're taking will not only stop working over time but will eventually make your blood pressure *increase.* This would undoubtedly scare you enough to call your doctor immediately to discuss other ways, medicinal or nonmedicinal, to manage your hypertension.

This exact scenario could occur if you're taking opioid or narcotic-based medications over a long period. Strange as it may sound, plenty of new research shows that these medications may make your symptoms *worse,* not better, over time. I have seen this happen over my twelve years of private practice.

But before we explore the ways that opioids can make a pain problem worse, let's take a look at what opioids are, what they do, how they work, and their possible side effects.

What Are Opioids?

Opioids are narcotic drugs that have been used for centuries to relieve pain. A narcotic is an addictive drug that reduces pain, induces sleep or stupor, and alters behavior and mood. Opioids contain opium or a derivative of opium, which is made from the dried juice of the unripe pods of the opium poppy. At the turn of the nineteenth century, morphine was isolated as the main alkaloid and active ingredient in opium and named after Morpheus, the Greek god of dreams. Soon after, the alkaloids codeine and papaverine were also discovered and isolated from opium. These and other raw materials found in opium are used to make many of the opioid drugs.

The use of opioid medications for the treatment of chronic pain became accepted practice in the mid 1990s, when numerous studies established their safety and efficacy and they received the support of several national organizations, including the American Academy of

Pain Medicine, the American Pain Society, and the Federation of State Medical Boards of the United States.

Here are some common opioid medications and their generic equivalents:

OPIOID MEDICATIONS

Generic Name	Trade Name	Indications
buprenorphine hydrochloride	Subutex, Suboxone	Treatment of opioid dependence and addiction
Codeine phosphate	Tylenol with codeine	Mild to moderate pain; cough suppressant
fentanyl patches	Duragesic	Persistent, moderate to severe chronic pain that cannot be managed by other means
fentanyl hydrochloride	Ionsys, Actiq	Short-term management of terminal illness
hydrocodone bitartrate	Vicodin, Norco, Lortab	Moderate to moderately severe pain
hydromorphone hydrochloride	Dilaudid	Acute severe pain
levorphanol tartrate	Levo-Dromoran	Moderate to severe pain; availability is limited
meperidine	Demerol	Moderate to severe pain; preoperative medication
methadone hydrochloride	Dolophine	Moderate to severe pain; detoxification treatment for opioid addiction
morphine sulfate (long- and short-acting)	MS Contin, Kadian, Avinza, Oramorph	Severe acute and severe chronic pain
oxycodone hydrochloride (long- and short-acting)	Oxycontin, Percocet, Endocet	Moderate to moderately severe pain
oxymorphone hydrochloride (long- and short-acting)	Opana	Moderate to severe pain in patients requiring continuous opioid treatment for an extended period
propoxyphene	Darvon, Darvocet	Mild pain
tramadol hydrochloride (long- and short-acting)	Ultram, Ultracet	Mild to moderate pain

Opioids, when properly used, can be very helpful medicines. Their pain-relieving capabilities make surgery and postoperative recovery much more tolerable. Likewise, short-acting and long-acting opioid pain medications have improved the quality of life for millions suffering from terminal illnesses such as cancer and AIDS. Opioids are a key component of modern medicine, and it's safe to say they are here to stay.

Beware the Side Effects—and Abuse

Despite being considered safe for the treatment of chronic pain by many experts and organizations, the opioids, like all medications, have side effects. Here are some of the common problems associated with the extended use of opioid-based painkillers:

- constipation
- sedation
- nausea
- sleep apnea
- confusion
- urinary retention
- hallucinations
- rebound headaches
- sexual dysfunction
- hormonal changes
- reduced REM sleep
- cognitive impairment

Then there's the problem of abuse. This is not just an adult problem. There has been a steady increase in the incidence of pain pill abuse by teenagers. In fact, the abuse of prescription pain medications is the fastest growing type of substance abuse among U.S. teens. These drugs are so easy for kids to get, these days they may find bowls filled with Vicodin and Oxycontin at their parties instead of pretzels and M&M's! A number of my patients with teenagers have discovered supplies of pain pills missing from their medicine cabinets. Some have even seen their kids extolling the virtues of their pain medications on YouTube videos!

The Pain Pill Paradox

Yet another downside to opioid use, apart from a hefty list of side effects and the very real possibility of abuse, is that they can actually *increase* the capacity to feel pain. I have seen this "pain-increasing power" when I've administered epidural cortisone injections. This procedure, which is often done to relieve symptoms such as subacute sciatica (low back and leg pain), is performed in a controlled environment with sedation and a local anesthetic in order to help patients feel more relaxed and comfortable. First the patient is given a sedative, then an injection of lidocaine to numb the skin, and finally the injection of cortisone into the epidural space of the spine.

This procedure is often painless or relatively comfortable. In fact, many patients are surprised at how easy it is—that is, unless they have been chronic users of opioid-based pain medications. Then it can be quite difficult. Many of these patients fidget and gasp from the discomfort, a much stronger reaction than that seen in those who don't take opioids, who usually don't stir at all. Once I begin injecting the cortisone, the opioid takers typically report a great deal more pain than those who are opioid free, and they may require supplemental doses of pain medicine and relaxants to help them get through the procedure.

Scientific research has revealed that this heightened sensitivity to pain is due to a prolonged exposure to opioid narcotics. I call this unsettling phenomenon the "pain pill paradox," but researchers have given it the more official-sounding name of *opioid-induced hyperalgesia* (OIH). Hyperalgesia means that the pain level is greater than expected. For example, while the squeezing action of a blood pressure cuff causes mild to moderate discomfort in the average person, it may cause excruciating pain in a person with hyperalgesia.

Am I really telling you that continuing to take some of the strongest pain medications in existence can actually make your chronic pain worse? Yes, I am! Would you take cholesterol medication if you knew it would eventually increase your cholesterol? How about sticking with a diabetes medication that would let your blood sugar zoom out of control? So why isn't anyone holding up a big red sign that says STOP? Or at least PROCEED WITH CAUTION? Think of the lessons learned in chapter 3. Do you think the pharmaceutical industry, which is a major sponsor of physician education, is anxious to let that cat out of the bag? My guess is not until they think they have found a product to counteract OIH.

I suspect denial is another reason why this research hasn't yet made a dent in doctors' prescription habits and patients' preferences. It seems it's hard for us to accept the fact that doing something widely believed to be right may not be so right after all. Unfortunately, when you have an office full of patients who want you to fix what ails them, it can be a lot more convenient to write prescriptions than work through the slower process of seeking out alternative solutions. This is often the case, regardless of whether we are talking about pain problems or other chronic conditions like heart disease and diabetes.

With OIH, the patient's pain is increased by the very medication he or she has been using to try to quell it. As his or her system becomes less responsive to the pain medications, the dose may be increased. This usually provides relief, which gives the impression that switching to a larger dose works. But the improvements don't last very long. Soon enough the pain returns at a heightened level (hyperalgesia). Thus the end result of the increase in medication is an increase in pain. It's a vicious cycle of pain, drugs, more pain, and more drugs.

An Important Distinction

Opioid-induced hyperalgesia is *not* the same phenomenon as

Tolerance, which develops when a medicine or other substance no longer has its desired effect. Tolerance doesn't imply that anything is getting worse.

Dependence, which describes how the body's chemistry changes or adapts to a medication so that stopping the medication would cause a withdrawal reaction.

Addiction, which implies that an individual cannot control his or her cravings for and use of a particular substance, resulting in potentially harmful behaviors.

David Clark, MD, a professor of anesthesia at Stanford University, coauthored a report on OIH for the American Society of Anesthesiologists in 2006. While acknowledging that scientists still can't predict who will develop this problem when exposed to narcotics, Clark made some interesting observations. Younger folks and those who have a history of addiction seem more prone to developing OIH, compared to elderly and never-addicted patients. More specifically, those who start taking opioid-based medications at age twenty or thirty are particularly likely to develop the clinical signs of hyperalgesia at some point. Thus if a person starts taking a medication such as morphine at a young age and continues over time, he or she will most likely experience changes in the way the brain cells respond to the morphine or other opioids.

Escaping the Pain Pill Paradox

In light of scientific evidence showing that long-term use of opioid pain pills often leads to other problems, I usually recommend that my patients transition to alternative methods to manage their chronic symptoms. For those of you focusing on living with chronic pain, as opposed to acute pain or pain from a malignancy, I suggest looking at this information differently. If drinking from polluted water makes you sick, you have the choice of continuing to drink from the same well and treating the diseases you get over and over again, or you can look for a water supply that is less contaminated. Every day I recommend to patients that they strongly consider transitioning off of opioid medications and developing alternative tools to manage their chronic symptoms.

I meet patients every day who don't want to stay on narcotic or opioid-type painkillers for the rest of their lives but have never been given any alternatives. Their doctors seem to offer them nothing but pills—more pills, different pills, new pills—because nobody seems to know what else to do. Once a feasible plan for leaving the pills behind is made available, most patients are happy to embrace it, even if they're afraid. And it *can* be a very scary step—but well worth it.

During their initial visit, I ask my patients a critical question: "Do you plan on taking these medications for the rest of your life?" Most are surprised by the question. But once they've had a few moments to collect their thoughts, they answer emphatically, "No, I don't!" This is often the first time a doctor has asked them this question and the first time they've discussed making a drastic change in their pain management regimen with an eye toward the future.

The immense problems caused by the pain pill paradox became apparent to my partner, John Massey, MD, and me when we started our first comprehensive pain program in 2001. We began this program in response to the large number of people we saw who were suffering from failed back syndrome. We constantly saw new patients who had undergone major spinal reconstructive surgery and were now in too much pain to move, despite taking potent dosages of narcotic painkillers. Most had been off work for years, and since the odds of going back to work are extremely low after being off for more than about six months, it seemed clear that most would remain disabled and unemployed. It goes without saying that most were also emotionally distraught.

At that time it was standard practice to prescribe opioid-based medications to fight the pain, so we typically did not ask patients in the program to stop taking their pain medications. Since it seemed as if many of our patients were not going to work again, we were just trying to help them as much as possible, and if that meant prescribing opioid-based meds, well, that's what it meant.

After a couple of years of trying to help these folks with their complex medical, social, and emotional problems, we came to a very clear realization: The patients in our program who took *none* of the typical narcotic painkillers while on our program not only did better, they were eventually able to go back to work. And going back to work after being off an average of five years beats odds greater than those in a Las Vegas casino! These folks also demonstrated a *motivation* that many of those taking painkillers couldn't match. This motivation influenced important areas of their lives, including work, exercise, and personal relationships.

Unfortunately, making drastic changes to medication intake isn't always easy. The symptoms of opioid withdrawal can include extreme anxiety, palpitations, sweating, agitation, diarrhea, and insomnia—all of which can linger. Gradually weaning off of high doses of narcotics can also be very taxing, as the withdrawal symptoms can drag on for periods longer than some can tolerate. This can be a lot to ask of someone who is also struggling with chronic pain and goes a long way toward explaining why many people are content to leave well enough alone.

Valuable Little Help in Combating Addiction

In 2004 we stumbled across a new medication called buprenorphine, which helps in the treatment of heroin addiction. Also known by the trade names Suboxone or Subutex, buprenorphine binds to opioid receptors in the body. This produces mild stimulating effects and simultaneously prevents opioids from binding to the receptors and producing their effects. Heroin addicts can take buprenorphine every day and get just enough of an effect to prevent withdrawal symptoms and cravings, but not enough of an effect to get high. And if they slip and use heroin again, the heroin can't compete with the buprenorphine for the opioid receptors, so it is negated. Studies show that as long as heroin addicts stay on buprenorphine, their rate of relapse is low.

Because it binds to the opioid receptors, buprenorphine can also be used to help patients get off of opioid-based narcotics. Since we began using it in our practice, buprenorphine has improved the lives of hundreds of our chronic pain patients. Giving up opioid-based narcotics helps them feel more clearheaded and more like their "old selves." In fact, many don't recognize the subtle cognitive effects their opioid medications produced until they've gotten them out of their systems. In most cases, as the haze lifts and the "old" personality starts to resurface, motivation isn't too far behind. While research is underway to pinpoint exactly how buprenorphine benefits chronic pain and impacts OIH, experience has taught me that it is an effective way to help patients transition off their opioid-based painkillers and lead more functional lives.

Don't Lose Your Perspective

There is no question that opioids have been a huge benefit to the practice of medicine. Undergoing most invasive surgeries would now be considered barbaric without narcotics as part of the anesthesia and postoperative recovery. Likewise, advances in creating novel opioid pain medications that are both quick acting and long acting has improved the dignity and quality of life for millions suffering from terminal illnesses such as cancer and AIDS. Unfortunately, opioids continue to be underutilized in patients with cancer, AIDS, and similar circumstances all over the world.

I remember meeting an acquaintance of my wife who, while living in one of the former Soviet states as a young girl, had her appendix removed. Instead of giving her a traditional anesthetic for the surgery, the doctors and caretakers held her down and poured some brandy and vodka down her throat before cutting out her appendix. This awful story reminds us how advances in pharmacology have made our lives easier and better. The problem I see every day is opioid overuse or abuse to the detriment of the people these medications are supposed to help.

I happen to enjoy drinking wine and find it a great complement to the pleasure of tasting and eating food. Ancient civilizations invented winemaking as far back as 6,000 B.C. It has long been used in Christian (Holy Communion) and Jewish (Kiddush) ceremonies and today is generally believed to have health benefits, when used in moderation. But when wine consumption goes from a glass with dinner to excessive overdrinking, it is no longer a health practice—it is alcoholism.

As we invent new drugs, devices, and technologies, we have to remember that they have the potential to create new problems, just as drinking three or four glasses of wine a day, as opposed to just one, can mean the difference between having a healthy heart and getting cirrhosis of the liver. I wrestle with problems each and every day that, unfortunately, were created by the overuse or misuse of treatments that our health care system embraces. Overdependence on opioid medications as a pain management tool seems to fall into this category. It is my job to take a step back, to look and see if what is going on is helping a patient go *forward* or *backward.*

Ending the long-term use of opioid medications can be a complex process; I don't recommend you take this upon yourself without first looking into the medical, social, community, and family resources available to assist you. However, I really *do* recommend that you reflect on what your "going forward plan" should look like. Imagine that you have optimum health. What does that look like, what does it mean to you, and how will you arrive at that point? What will be the state of your physical and emotional health in a year, in ten years, in twenty years? Do you see yourself still in pain and taking medicine, or do you see yourself healthy and happy without medicine? What changes do you need to make in order to achieve the physical and emotional well-being you want and deserve?

Suppose I told you that when you hit a certain age, say seventy-five, I was going to give you the body of a seventy-five-year-old that had never been taken care of. You would most certainly protest. Don't give that same uncared-for seventy-five-year-old body to yourself. And don't expect some magical medicine to come down the pike *and solve all your health problems for you later.* Start planning now so that you can live the next ten, twenty, thirty, even fifty years to their fullest. Doing so is a big step toward regaining control and taking charge of your life.

CHAPTER 5

The Verdict Is In: What Evidence-Based Medicine Says about Treating Pain

Modern medicine has amassed a lot of knowledge about managing pain. Unfortunately, we're not particularly efficient when it comes to spreading that knowledge among physicians who treat people suffering from various forms of pain. As a matter of fact, the best pain management information we have is routinely overlooked by the majority of health care providers, who usually just want to find the pain generator and fix it—right now!

Pain medicine or *pain management* has been a recognized medical specialty for less than twenty years. It's a necessary specialty, for chronic pain is a disease of our modern era, much like coronary artery disease and type 2 diabetes. Now that we can usually avoid death from infections that used to wipe out whole societies, thanks to hand washing and antibiotics, we find ourselves hanging around much longer. That's wonderful; but what happens when we're in pain for much of that time?

Here is an example of my point: I saw a very nice gentleman in my office the other day. He is fifty years old and has been a construction worker all of his life. Now, thirty years of heavy physical work, day in and day out, takes its toll on a body. He has aches and pains all over the place, including irritated nerves around both his neck and lower back. Financially he feels he must continue to work up to seven days a week, and he doesn't know any other type work to even consider at this point. During Ancient Roman times, the average male seldom lived past thirty years old; no doubt building those aqueducts was hard work. However, my middle-aged patient has a good chance of living another thirty years or more. Managing pain is now a very important health issue that he will need to deal with for decades to come. And he will need help doing so, which is why the specialty of pain medicine or pain management is so necessary.

Thankfully, John Bonica, MD, developed the key concepts of modern pain management. He became an impassioned anesthesiologist, dedicated to alleviating the human suffering that doctors from other specialties tended to ignore. While serving as head of an Army hospital during World War II, he realized that the time-honored concept of having a single physician or therapist to treat chronic pain was generally ineffective, for it was better understood and managed when a team of complementary providers worked together, each offering his or her special insights and therapies. Thanks to this early understanding and his later pioneering efforts, Bonica became the father of the multidisciplinary model of chronic pain management. With his passing in 1994, he left behind five decades of remarkable work that created a new specialty devoted to treating acute and chronic pain, which is now known as pain medicine or pain management.

Evidence-Based Medicine: A New Approach

The pain management specialty has been around for two decades, so you might think we should have the problem licked by now. Unfortunately we don't, partially because medicine continues to be practiced in a highly individual way. Despite the fact that medical schools across the country all use the same basic textbooks to teach future physicians; that doctors across the country read many of the same studies and articles published in the *Journal of the American Medical Association,* the *New England Journal of Medicine, Lancet,* and other major medical journals; and that doctors across the country attend conferences that feature discussions on prevailing concepts and approaches, the practice of medicine is still highly personal. By that I mean there is no national consensus regarding the best way to handle many diseases and conditions, from heart attacks to pregnancy to pain. You would expect the Cesarean section rate, for example, to be about the same from coast to coast, with only minor variations to account for the average age, general health, or other factors of the mothers-to-be. You would also expect the number of back surgeries, coronary bypasses, prescriptions for antidepressants, use of "clot-busting" drugs for strokes, recommendations to lose weight, and just about everything else doctors do to be about the same from California to Maine, with slight differences to accommodate variations in local populations. In other words, you'd think that people going to their doctors with Disease X would receive more or less the same treatment, no matter where they live.

This is not the case. Rates for certain surgeries, medication prescriptions, referrals to physical therapy, and other factors vary widely from city to city and state to state, because doctors base their diagnoses and treatment decisions on a combination of their own knowledge, personal experience, and local practice—that is, what other doctors in the community do.

While experience is a marvelous teacher, it can be misleading; it is, by definition, limited to what one person has observed and concluded. But is every doctor insightful and dispassionate enough to make arm's-length observations of his or her own work and draw the appropriate conclusions? For example, a particular doctor might believe that she gets great results using Drug X, but her opinion might be skewed by the fact that some of her patients who did *not* respond to Drug X drifted off to other doctors, while others told her what they thought she wanted to hear rather than risk offending her. Similarly, the local practice may be a helpful guide, but it is subject to the same kinds of biases seen in individual practice, though on a larger scale. In general, doctors tend to follow their experiences and stick with what they *believe* works.

Alarmed by disparities in the treatments offered and results obtained around the country, a small body of researchers and physicians began to promote the idea that everything physicians do should be based on sound scientific evidence—that is, evidence-based medicine (EBM). While there would always be a place for experience (which would help physicians fine-tune their application of scientifically proven techniques), the goal of EBM is to provide physicians with the best available *evidence* to enable them to make conscientious and effective decisions about treatments.

To illustrate this concept, let's look at the use of chicken soup as a remedy for a seasonal cold. Tradition—and your own personal experience—dictates that the soup be cooked according to your grandmother's special recipe and eaten in plentiful amounts. As a result you should get back on your feet in no time. EBM experts would carefully analyze the outcomes of chicken soup use. They would look at numerous published scientific studies on chicken soup, carefully considering the types of viruses it was used for, as well as the ages of the patients, degree of sickness, and other factors. Next they would compare the ingredients in your grandmother's soup to the ingredients in your neighbor's, provided your neighbor has published her recipe and results. They would look at how many days people have runny noses when they eat the soup compared to the number of days they have runny noses when they don't eat the soup. Maybe they would compare the number of missed workdays between chicken soup eaters and non–chicken soup eaters. Certain conflicts are bound to arise, of course. For example, one published study might say both groups miss the same number of days, while twelve others say the soup eaters miss an average of two days less. Our experts would reconcile that conflicting information by analyzing the data. Once the designated EBM gurus had carefully analyzed as much scientific information as they could find on chicken soup, they would publish their results and devise guidelines on its use. (By the way, even if EBM fails to find that your grandmother's chicken soup is an effective treatment for the common cold, that doesn't necessarily mean it is without merit. It might actually work better than anything else, but if it hasn't been subjected to enough rigorous scientific study, the experts won't recommend for or against it.)

Over the last five years, EBM has received a lot of attention from multiple sources. The federal government, for example, is trying to figure out how to reward doctors for following EBM guidelines in an effort to control the costly Medicare system. And an organization called the Cochrane Collaboration, named for Scottish epidemiologist Archie Cochrane, has become a leading developer and a repository of EBM studies. The Cochrane Collaboration is devoted to "improving healthcare decision-making globally, through systematic reviews of the effects of healthcare intervention."[5] The results of their studies are published on the Cochrane Library Web site, a large database of systematic reviews of different treatments. Its information is provided free to residents in several countries, including the United Kingdom.

A number of analytical think tanks promote best practice guidelines in health care, as do articles and guidelines published in the medical literature, but when was the last time your doctor talked to you about evidence-based medicine? Unfortunately, there is an excellent chance that your doctor is still treating you on the basis of personal experience and local practice habits.

The Pain Verdict

At this point you are probably wondering what EBM says about treating chronic pain. As it turns out, several different EBM reviews have come to the same conclusion: The best approach to the treatment of chronic pain is a *comprehensive interdisciplinary pain program in which professionals from a variety of complementary disciplines work* together, usually under one roof, in an integrated manner to achieve common treatment goals for their patients.

Yes, we live in a very technologically advanced age, with regular breakthroughs in pharmacology, genetics, and more, and the best I can come up with is a concept that was invented over fifty years ago by someone named Bonica, a doctor you only heard of a few minutes ago. That's right. The evidence all points to the idea that a team of health experts working together is superior to a single doctor or to a series of uncoordinated treatments from different doctors and therapists.

5 "The Cochrane Collaboration." Accessible at http://www.cochrane.org/. Viewed July 18, 2009.

A number of comprehensive EBM reviews of chronic pain performed over the last several years all support the use of special pain programs (which I will explain in a bit). These reviews were published in prominent journals such as the *Journal of the American Medical Association, Pain,* and the *Journal of Pain.* The most recent and comprehensive review was conducted by two highly regarded academicians (two very smart persons who do this type of thing for a living): Robert Gatchel, from the University of Texas, and Akiko Okifuji, from the University of Utah. Gatchel and Okifuji reported a number of interesting findings after conducting an extensive review and critique of the available information from around the world. They clearly noted that when interdisciplinary pain programs were compared to conventional treatments or surgeries, the interdisciplinary programs came out ahead on key parameters including the following:

- Levels of pain: This refers to a patient's self-report of pain, for there are no objective measures of pain. Someone might say, "I have fewer flare-ups" or "My pain is less intense now."
- Function: This includes things like being better able to take care of themselves, clean their house, do their gardening, and walk.
- Health care utilization: This includes things such as fewer doctor's visits, fewer tests, and fewer health care resources needed after treatment.
- Cost: It costs less to treat a patient in an interdisciplinary program than in customary treatment.
- Medication use: Patients tended to require fewer pain medications following treatment.
- Return-to-work rates: A key outcome measurement that remained consistently positive in all the studies.

The Evidence Is In

In their concluding comments, Robert Gatchel and Akiko Okifuji summarize chronic pain treatment nicely: "Chronic pain is a ubiquitous medical condition. Traditionally, pain has been conceptualized as a symptom reflecting an underlying pathology. Many chronic pain cases, however, fail to fit into such a category, rather manifesting as multisystem illnesses that significantly compromise major parts of the patient's functional life. For these cases, the standard medical approach or medication management does not seem to provide much relief. The only therapeutic approach that has shown efficacy and cost-effectiveness is a CPP [chronic pain program], with functional restoration as a primary goal. Indeed, based on the growing number of randomized, controlled trials from different clinical research centers in the United States and other countries, there is unequivocal evidence for the effectiveness of CPPs. There is now more evidence-based research documenting this effectiveness than for any other medical treatment approach."[6]

What Is a Comprehensive Interdisciplinary Pain Program?

Soon after my partner and I started our practice, other doctors began sending us lots of patients who had just undergone extensive spine surgeries. These folks frequently had multiple problems: trouble moving due to severe pain, the economic stress of being off work, anxiety about their futures, and depression. In addition, they were often taking lots of strong medications every few hours.

My partner and I knew about the medical aspects of pain management, but we also realized that there was a lot more to managing chronic pain than prescribing pills or doing nerve blocks. We enlisted nutritionists to help our patients control their weight and eat more healthfully, psychologists to help them grapple with emotional issues, and physical therapists to teach them how to use their bodies despite their pain. We were open to all sorts of ideas. For

---

6   Gatchel, R.J., Okifuji, A. Evidence-based scientific data documenting the treatment and cost-effectiveness of comprehensive pain programs for chronic nonmalignant pain. *J. Pain.* 2006 Nov; 7(11):779–93.

example, having seen how helpful art therapy was as a tool for handling grief in cancer care, I was keen to try it out on chronic pain patients. One of the first people we hired was a counselor who had special training as an art therapist. As we brought each health care provider on board, we insisted that he or she share our commitment to the team approach.

Our program evolved as we learned more, and today it is highly structured and intensive. Our patients spend each day going from class to class, in small group settings, learning from a team of providers. This is where the *interdisciplinary* part comes in: different specialists working together in an integrated manner. Bringing together distinct and unique perspectives offers us a greater opportunity to understand and treat the whole person. Each specialist complements the others, making the experience for the patient greater than the sum of the parts. *(Multidisciplinary* care resembles interdisciplinary treatment, but the team members may not all work in the same office space, with the same level of integration among each other.)

One of the primary benefits of interdisciplinary programs is that they help correct or eliminate unfortunate habits that can prolong or worsen chronic pain, such as

- Inactivity: A common side effect of pain that can make things hurt even more.
- Frequent doctor visits: Too many chefs can ruin the stew.
- Taking medications every day: At some point, the medical side effects may outweigh the benefits.
- Avoiding social contacts who are not related to medical treatments: This only makes depression worse.
- Anger: Negative thoughts can cause mood changes that worsen pain symptoms.
- Waiting for someone else to find the answer: Successful patients participate in the quest for better health.
- Fearful thoughts about getting worse: These scare you into interfering with your own recovery.

- Missing work: Pain is one the leading causes of missed work time.
- Spending hours on the Internet looking for help or just plain looking: This takes away from exercise, fresh air, having fun, and other more healthy pursuits.

In my highly structured, comprehensive, interdisciplinary program, the way chronic pain patients spend their time is changed dramatically. Here's how:

- They go from avoiding physical activities to exercising one to two hours every day. They are exposed to traditional gym routines as well as to movements associated with Eastern cultures, such as tai chi. Most people make dramatic gains in their physical capabilities, including their ability to walk, lift, and carry, as well as improvements in body mechanics and usage.
- They learn how to relax, meditate, and relieve stress.
- They learn to change the way they think about things that might not be helpful, or may even be disruptive, to their well-being.
- They can take art therapy classes and learn other techniques to boost the creative side of their brains and open new lines of communication.
- They gain access to specialists who can help them find jobs, volunteer opportunities, and other meaningful activities.
- They work with their families. Sometimes family members take classes with the patient, while other times they go to classes designed to help them cope with the stresses of living with a chronic pain patient.

A well-designed comprehensive pain program also offers participants plenty of *contact time,* or time spent with doctors and therapists. And studies show that greater amounts of contact time lead to better results.

I've seen many people suffering from chronic pain turn their lives around after enrolling in a comprehensive interdisciplinary pain program that helps them use medicines wisely and sparingly, utilize physical and psychological therapies, master techniques of stress reduction and relaxation, learn to eat healthfully, and change the way they think about themselves. I've seen them learn to manage their pain, regain control of their lives, and rediscover the joy of life.

But I've also seen—and continue to see—many people who are trapped in chronic pain by a health care system that still emphasizes having either a single doctor or a series of isolated, non-communicating health care specialists "fix" the problem with powerful drugs and surgeries, right now!

Are You in Control?

Take a moment to reflect on **control.**

Do you feel as though you are in control of your pain? Or is it the other way around? Is your pain dictating what you can do physically each day? Are you avoiding get-togethers with friends because of your pain? Have you given up on some hobbies or stopped exercising? Do you rely on your doctor's prescriptions as your only hope for feeling better?

Now is the time to begin regaining control of your life by identifying which parts of your life are being manipulated or hampered by your pain and developing a winning plan to overcome it. A good way to start is to choose a few things that you *can* do each day—and then do them so you have some sense of control, a feeling that you are back in the driver's seat. You'll find ideas to help you do this in the upcoming chapters.

Create Your Own Program

The evidence is clear: Fixating on a pain generator, focusing on heavy-duty medicines and surgeries, and attempting to "fix" chronic pain immediately is not likely to relieve your chronic pain. In fact, doing so may set you up for years or even decades of escalating pain as you stumble from one problem to the next and one doctor to the next, never finding relief for your growing list of pains and other problems.

The best approach is a comprehensive interdisciplinary pain management program. Unfortunately, millions of chronic pain patients are not participating in such programs. The fact that you're reading this book suggests that you are not, and you are not satisfied with the treatment you're receiving. If that's the case, keep reading. In the chapters to come I'll show you how you can adopt many of the principles of a comprehensive interdisciplinary pain management program on your own or with some help from your physician and other health care providers. By adopting many of the principles and practices we've successfully used in our program, there's an excellent chance you can reverse your downward spiral and start to put your pain in its place!

Can You See a Great Future?

When I first see new patients, I ask them questions like, "How do you plan on managing your pain for the next forty years?" and "Do you plan on taking those medications for the rest of your life?" Over the next few visits, I try to develop a plan that will not only help them get through the next day, but will last a lifetime. Invariably they let me know that nobody has ever asked them questions like that or suggested making such a plan, and they are onboard and willing to make the changes that will point them toward a better future.

Perhaps they've never thought about making these changes because they didn't have a *vision* of what they wanted life to look like. If they are in my office, chances are they want to make big changes, but they don't yet know which ones or how to implement them. I often tell them about my financial planner, who coached me into developing a vision of what I wanted my life to look like as I grew older. It became his job to figure out how I was going to pay for all of the fun and games I imagined enjoying right up to the end of life. I recommend you formulate the same type of vision for yourself and start to nourish your body, mind, and soul as you begin your journey.

The truths of the first five chapters have taught us important facts, theories, discoveries, biases, and misnomers in chronic pain management. This information makes it easier for us to grow in the direction we all want to go—toward control. We are now closer to having that clean slate I alluded to earlier. Since change starts from within, Part II, "Think," will prepare you for that process by helping you better understand your stress, emotions, thoughts, and fears. You will learn how each of these is connected and of the crippling effect chronic pain can have on them. After gaining this awareness, you will be ready for the breakthroughs awaiting you in Part III.

THINK

CHAPTER 6

Stress: The Silent Killer

Imagine that instead of being a sophisticated member of the *Homo sapiens* species, you are a zebra roaming the Serengeti region of Africa. Your typical day involves waking up, sipping some organic pond water, and munching on grass, which is your favorite dish. Now let's suppose that in the midst of your blissful day you suddenly see a lion coming your way, and she thinks that *you* look like *her* favorite dish. What happens next? You run like mad! Your legs pump as hard and as fast as you can possibly make them go. Your whole body feels tense and tight. You keep moving in this fashion until you have safely gotten away from the predator who was moments ago nipping at your heels with sharp teeth and an empty stomach.

At this point if you weren't really a zebra, you would likely be quite shaken by what just happened. I mean you were almost a lion's lunch! You would probably run and rerun through your head what just happened. Images of a very scary lion chasing you would remain in your thoughts. You might start to feel afraid that the lion may come back. This anxiety would keep you up at night, and you would avoid leaving the house as much as possible because you'd be terrified of experiencing a similar struggle for survival. In other words, you would find yourself not letting go of the memories of what happened, and this would modify your behavior.

The zebra, on the other hand, responds to the threat with a series of genetically programmed physiological reactions that are necessary for its survival. Then once the "great escape" becomes "mission accomplished," the zebra goes back to grazing for food and frolicking with its pals. It's able to let go of the memories of the stressful event and move on. If we humans could act more like zebras when under stress, we'd be a lot happier and healthier! This wonderful concept comes to us courtesy of Robert M. Sapolsky in his easy-to-read book on stress, *Why Zebras Don't Get Ulcers.* I often recommend this valuable book to new patients.

What is Stress?

Stress is defined as "the experience of a challenging event." That event can be physical, mental, emotional, or a combination of two or all three. Being chased by a lion is, of course, a physical challenge, while friction in a personal relationship is an emotional challenge. Here's another example of an emotional challenge: You've been assigned to work with a difficult coworker on a special project, and your boss has hinted that if that project is unsuccessful you may lose your job. You've got to get along with this person even though you find yourself grinding your teeth and suffering from a pounding headache every time you talk to him.

A mental challenge, in contrast, involves intense thought work or doing tasks that require mental concentration, especially under time pressure. For example, if you were given ten minutes to complete ten calculus problems, you'd probably find your heart rate soaring, your temperature rising, and sweat beading up on your forehead.

The point of these examples is that the reactions created by physical, emotional, and mental challenges are almost identical. So you can end up feeling very much the same whether a lion is chasing you, you're arguing with a colleague, or you're doing heavy-duty calculus. The experience of pain, too, creates an internal stress reaction, leading to the same physiologic changes. Part III will teach you techniques that reduce stress and combat the negative effects it can have on your body.

Fight or Flight

The physiological reaction that occurs inside each of us when faced with a stressful event is called the *fight-or-flight response.* Our bodies quickly go through a chain reaction of events that enables us to survive the threat by making us ready to either fight off the challenge or run like mad to get away from it. The fight-or-flight response is not unique to human beings; other mammals behave similarly. This was the adaptive trait that the zebra used to outrun that lion. We will see later in the chapter that our brains take this primitive survival mechanism further than other mammals, leading to problems associated with stress, like ulcers.

The fight-or-flight response works like this: The body needs more energy—and it needs it fast—to do the extra work required to either fight or flee. This means the heart must pump more blood, because blood carries glucose (the body's fuel) and oxygen to the body's tissues.

The heart beats more forcefully during the fight-or-flight response after it receives commands from the brain to pump harder and faster. This helps to quickly move more blood to the tissues so they can burn more energy right away. The amount of blood the heart pumps each minute is known as *cardiac output*. (Technically speaking, cardiac output is figured by multiplying the volume pumped by the heart with each beat, by the heart rate, or number of beats per minute.) Increases in cardiac output usually lead to increases in blood pressure.

The lungs also do their part to deliver more energy to the tissues. To keep up with the increased demand for oxygen, the breathing rate increases so the body can quickly absorb more oxygen into the blood. Breathing faster also means the lungs can get rid of waste products like carbon dioxide, which are created from all that running around. As the body burns more fuel, more waste products are created and need to be eliminated, just like a car needs to blow off exhaust. When carbon dioxide builds up as a waste product, the lungs get rid of it by breathing it out into the air.

The extra blood pumped by the heart is sent to the brain and muscles, the tissues that need it most, while less blood goes to the immune system and organs like the stomach, kidneys, and liver. This makes sense when you consider that the goal is to run as fast as possible or throw knockout punches. Later, when things have calmed down, the body can focus on things like digesting food or chasing down bacteria.

The extra blood that goes to the brain is directed to specific areas that govern activity, such as the brain stem and the limbic system. The brain stem is responsible for involuntary activities like breathing and heart rate. The limbic system deals with emotions; thus you can get mad, angry, or excited at the same time that everything else is going on.

As these changes in circulation occur, the body's physiology also changes. There is a slowdown in activity in the bowels and pelvis, which can bring about cramping, constipation, and a lack of erectile activity (if that happens to be an issue at that particular time). Constriction of the small blood vessels can cause cold, clammy hands. Muscles in the neck, shoulders, and jaw tighten up, which may trigger headaches. The nervous system becomes more sensitive to stimulation: Noises sound louder, light looks brighter, and smells become more pungent. Increased sweating allows the body to stay cool even as it burns more fuel than usual. Many people feel the fight-or-flight response as "butterflies in the stomach," that feeling you get when you are about to go onstage or tee off at the first hole of a golf tournament.

The Physiology of Stress

This lightning-fast reaction to a challenging event involves at least three different body systems: the nervous system, the endocrine system, and the immune system.

A part of the nervous system called *the autonomic nervous system* is heavily involved in the fight-or-flight response. The autonomic nervous system manages involuntary activities like respiration, heartbeat, and digestion. In short, it takes care of the things necessary to survival that we don't have to think about, like body temperature. The autonomic nervous system has special receptors in the skin that sense changes in temperature. If we become too warm or cold, it instructs the blood vessels to open or close, controlling the amount of heat released through the skin. Other nerves governed by the autonomic nervous system tell sweat glands when to secrete fluid to cool the body down, helping to regulate core temperature with a high level of precision.

The autonomic nervous system has two branches: the *sympathetic nervous system* (SNS) and the *parasympathetic nervous system* (PNS). These two opposing systems exist in a delicate balance. The SNS is activated during stressful events and triggers the fight-or-flight response. In just a few seconds, it zips out messages to organs such as the heart, telling it to beat faster, and to the intestines, telling them to contract more slowly. The SNS is also responsible for constricting blood vessels to direct the flow of blood to the muscles and the brain and for stimulating sweat glands to induce perspiration.

The PNS has the opposite effect. It brings on a state of relaxation and helps conserve energy, directing the heart and breathing rates to slow down, while stimulating the intestines to push food through more quickly. When the PNS is more active than the SNS, we generally feel calmer and less stressed.

The endocrine system—composed of hormones, glands, and target sites—triggers a cascade of events almost immediately after the body detects a stressful event. The word *hormone*—from a Greek word that means "to set in motion"—refers to a chemical substance produced in the body that controls and regulates the activity of specific cells or organs. Glands are the organs that produce the hormones, while the target sites are the places in the body where the hormones exert their effects.

To demonstrate how this works, let's look at the adrenal glands. The adrenal glands sit on top of the kidneys and manufacture several hormones, including epinephrine (also known as adrenaline). Epinephrine is produced in response to physical or mental stress and stimulates an increase in blood pressure, metabolic rate, and blood glucose concentration, while speeding the heart's action. Once it's secreted by the adrenal glands, epinephrine circulates through the bloodstream until it reaches a target site, such as the heart, where it delivers the message to beat faster and stronger.

The Dangers of Too Much Stress

The many changes that occur in the body in preparation to fight or flee can save lives. If overdone, however, this process can become dangerous, for the brain has its own glands, including the hypothalamus and pituitary, that can keep the "stress dialogue" in play for a long time.

When stress occurs too frequently, the levels of epinephrine and other hormones in the blood begin to rise. When the amount of another hormone, cortisol, becomes elevated, it can cause harmful inflammatory reactions in the brain, heart, and other vital tissues. It can also increase blood sugar, which over time can cause the body to become resistant to insulin and set the stage for diabetes. Increased cortisol levels have other dangerous consequences, too, including protein breakdown, which causes muscle wasting and atrophy; sodium and water retention; increased blood pressure; and a reduction in bone density, which can contribute to the unhealthy thinning of the bones known as osteoporosis.

Chronic exposure to cortisol and other stress hormones can also suppress the immune system, the body's special "police force" that identifies and destroys bacteria, viruses, and other "invaders" and also keeps cancer from growing or spreading within the tissues. A weakening of the immune system can open the door to a host of problems—from annoying colds that linger too long, to outright diseases such as pneumonia, to cancers that grow unchecked.

When stress becomes chronic, hormones that were at lower levels during calmer times can become prominent and throw things "out of whack," hormonally speaking. What's tolerable for the short term can become dangerous over the long haul. And the longer the brain feels challenged, the longer it will direct the adrenal glands to secrete extra cortisol and otherwise keep the pot boiling.

Excess Stress Equals Inflammation

As we have seen, stress upsets homeostasis, or the balance within the body. This, in turn, leads to negative changes, including inflammation, which comes from the Latin word that means "to set on fire."

Celsus, an ancient Roman physician, described four classic signs of inflammation: redness, pain, heat, and swelling. We need look no further than a sunburn to see what the Roman doctor meant. The skin turns red, is painful to touch, and feels warm and swollen. This is the body's way of handling the injury and eventually removing the damaged skin cells. So even though inflammation is helpful because it destroys invading germs or harmful substances within the body, healthy body tissue can be damaged in the process. The body tries to repair the damage, but is not always 100 percent successful.

The inflammation process starts with increased blood flow to the problem area, which may be a cut, infection, burn, and so on. Small blood vessels open wide, or dilate, to make sure immune system cells and mediators of inflammation can get to the area. Cytokines, chemicals produced by the immune cells to help orchestrate the attack, are released to help fight the enemy. As more and more defending cells and substances arrive on the scene, the tissue begins to look redder and more swollen. The blood vessels also become more "leaky," which means they develop pores to allow the immune cells and cytokines to squeeze through so they can reach their target. In the case of sunburn, the skin at this point might be so swollen, red, and painful that you wouldn't even want to touch it.

Sunburn or a swollen knee produces the kind of inflammation that you can see with the naked eye. But there is also a kind of inflammation that occurs internally, on a microscopic level, that can become chronic and pose a danger at certain critical locations within the body. Chronic inflammation can cause quite a bit of tissue destruction, followed by repeated attempts by the body to repair what has been destroyed. During the repair process the body creates scar tissue in the damaged areas, a process called fibrosis. The scar tissue is necessary to patch things back together, but scarred body parts do not work as well as healthy parts.

You can see this happen with a heart attack, or myocardial infarction. If you were to examine under a microscope a sample of the damaged heart tissue a few months after the attack, you would see that scar tissue has formed. This damaged part of the heart cannot pump blood as effectively as it did when it had viable muscle cells. But it doesn't take a catastrophe like a heart attack to damage tissue and provoke scar tissue. Repeated jolts of stress, along with the massive changes in chemistry that result, can keep the inflammation fires burning within the body. This puts many organs at risk of being damaged, repaired but scarred, and unable to work quite as well as they once did.

Stress and the Brain

Even the brain is not protected from inflammation. Chronic stress and the resulting chronic inflammation ultimately damage brain cells, just as they do other cells in the body. How that damage plays out depends on the part of the brain that is damaged. For example, if the damage occurs in the hippocampus, an area of the brain involved with memory and learning, it may impair a patient's ability to learn new material or remember things. For as long as I have been practicing medicine, patients have been telling me that it became much more difficult to remember things after they developed chronic pain. It was as if their minds just didn't work the way they used to, and they had to struggle with short-term memory, like remembering what they did an hour ago. While there can be many different factors contributing to forgetfulness, chronic stress most certainly plays a part.

What's more, research has shown that Alzheimer's disease correlates with evidence of chronic inflammation around the brain cells. Small proteins known as amyloid beta proteins clump around cells in the brain and cause inflammation. This inflammation causes brain cell atrophy, cognitive impairment, and Alzheimer's disease—

one of the saddest diseases in existence. Unfortunately, there is no cure for Alzheimer's disease and other forms of chronic dementia. The only strategy is to avoid getting these diseases in the first place (more on that in chapter 18).

The Link between Chronic Inflammation and Chronic Pain

We now know that chronic inflammation is associated with some of our most common medical problems, including diabetes, cardiovascular disease, cancer, arthritis, and Alzheimer's disease. Yet another inflammation-related disease is metabolic syndrome. Caused in part by inflammation, metabolic syndrome is a precursor to life-threatening diseases like coronary heart disease, cardiovascular disease, and diabetes. Among other things, it's characterized by abdominal obesity, mildly elevated blood sugar, increased triglycerides, insulin resistance, and inflammation. Believe it or not, experts think that about one in four American adults have metabolic syndrome! In other words, about a quarter of us who don't yet have a serious chronic disease are about to develop one.

Chronic inflammation is also linked to chronic pain in a cause-and-effect relationship. Let me explain: Inflammation is a key component of painful diseases such as rheumatoid arthritis, in which the body's own antibodies attack tissues in the joints, causing inflammation and swelling. Inflammation can erupt from the stress caused by painful chronic conditions such as migraine headaches or low back pain. To put it simply, there is a direct connection between chronic pain and the development of a stress reaction, which in turn increases the likelihood of chronic inflammation. And, as we have seen, chronic inflammation is an important factor in the development of metabolic syndrome, diabetes, heart disease, obesity, and other deadly diseases. It's no wonder that stress—thanks to its by-product, inflammation—has been called the *"silent killer."*

Stress is intimately linked to chronic pain; that's why I tell my patients that one of the best "medicines" for their pain is learning how to control their stress, which I'll talk about in Part III.

A Final Word on Waste Management

Life can be "messy," even inside the body. For example, as our cells create the energy they need to function, they give off by-products called free radicals. These free radicals, if not cleaned up, can cause inflammation and harm the very cells that created them as well as other cells. This harmful process is known as oxidative stress.

Within our cells are small energy-producing engines known as mitochondria, which give off harmful free radicals as waste products. Antioxidants help clean free radicals from the mitochondria so that they can continue to burn fuel efficiently and keep the cells healthy. Certain foods provide bountiful supplies of these helpful antioxidants, and we will learn about them in chapter 15. But excess free radicals, which may come from a poor diet, environmental toxins, and stress, can overwhelm the mitochondria's ability to protect itself and function properly. When free radical levels rise too high, the cells become overrun with inflammation, and this, as we have seen, can lead to chronic medical problems. Eating a healthy diet and taking supplements helps provide your body with the antioxidants it needs to prevent inflammation and the resulting diseases from occurring—and so does reducing your stress levels.

Our bodies are equipped with detoxification mechanisms designed to eliminate waste products such as excess free radicals. While each cell in the body can eliminate some toxins, the liver is the primary organ for this process. But when our systems become overloaded with excessive levels of toxins, pain and fatigue levels can rise and brain function can suffer. Stress and the inflammation it triggers can wear out or overwhelm our internal waste management system and lead to this increase in toxins. Therefore, reducing stress is a form of preventive medicine.

Helpful Measurements

If you let yourself get out of shape, your metabolism will slow down. You will burn fuel more slowly and less efficiently because your mitochondria won't work as well. Interval training, for example, has been shown to stimulate the production of more mitochondria inside the cells. Interval training is a type of exercise where you alternate periods of intense aerobic activity with brief periods of rest. Sprinting fifty yards and then walking fifty yards on a repeated basis is an example of interval training.

There is a way to measure how fit you are, although it is not commonly available to those of us who are not Olympic athletes in training. The test, known as maximal oxygen consumption (VO2), measures how well body tissues utilize oxygen when exercising. (There are specialty health centers around the country that have the equipment and staff to measure your VO2, if you have the means to go there and have it done.) What's the stress-VO2 connection? Stress causes a buildup of wastes in the body, and this nasty accumulation can interfere with your ability to perform aerobic exercise. VO2 measures your exercise capacity. So if you cannot exercise well, it may be because your body is flooded with stress-induced waste products. This means that the VO2 is not just a measure of your ability to utilize oxygen, but it is also an indirect measure of your overall health.

Another test, which is accessible to most of us around the United States, is a blood test that measures C-reactive protein (CRP), a protein that is released from liver and fat cells. The higher the CRP level, the higher the level of inflammation in the body. In the face of acute inflammation, CRP can rise in a matter of hours to many thousands of times the normal level. Measuring CRP levels is a helpful tool to gauge inflammation at a micro level that can't be seen or felt. However, it does not tell you where the inflammation is coming from. If your doctor knows where the problem area is, then he or she can monitor its progress over time.

Protecting our most valuable resource—our brain—from the harmful effects of stress and inflammation is an important part of a winning pain management plan, as you will see in the next two chapters.

CHAPTER 7
The Brain in Pain

Maintaining a healthy brain can be a lot like farming. Growing produce is really a simple process, but there are many little nuances that determine the fate of the crops each year. First of all, farmers need soil and seeds, and they must use them properly. They must *plant* cucumber seeds in order to harvest cucumbers and not watermelon. And if they don't plant anything, all they can expect are some random weeds. They will reap what they sow.

There must also be good soil in which the fruits and vegetables can take root. It must have the right kinds and amounts of nutrients if the specific crop is to develop to its fullest potential. The *type* of soil is important, too. The best soil for growing cabernet sauvignon wine grapes is not necessarily the best soil for raising chardonnay grapes.

Of course farmers must also water their plants, or else many, if not all, will die. The environment is also important, for each type of plant needs a special mix of sunshine and seasonal changes. Too much or too little rain can ruin a crop. Farmers must also tend to their grounds so they work more efficiently, tilling or turning the soil to provide a better growing environment.

The great news is that if we adopt these simple farming philosophies to our bodies, we can change the way chronic pain impacts our lives in powerful ways.

Neurogenesis
The billions of cells in the human brain are similar to cells throughout the body in that they are the basic "action units" of the organ. The brain's busy action units are also known as *neurons.* Scientists used to think that the brain was fixed for adults, meaning it was not capable of changing or regenerating itself. There were a certain number of neurons present at birth, and when one was seri-

ously damaged or destroyed, perhaps by a stroke, it would never be repaired or replaced.

We now know that is not true, that the brain is a very dynamic organ, even later in life. Yes, I *am* suggesting that aging, decaying, shrinking brains have the ability to create new cells and thus regenerate themselves to some degree. This assertion is backed by scientific evidence conducted over the last ten years, which has debunked the myth that human brains stop creating new nerve tissue after birth. Fred Gage, PhD, a research scientist at the Salk Institute in La Jolla, California, demonstrated that *neurogenesis*—the creation of new neurons—takes place in adult brains. And other research is currently being conducted to help us understand precisely how this occurs, exactly what it means for brain health, and by extension, what it means for the health of the entire body. This is one of the most exciting bits of news for chronic pain management, yet nobody in my field seems to be talking about it!

A dynamic, malleable, and ever-evolving brain can play an important role in managing health, including the management of chronic pain. Unfortunately, doctors everywhere are ignoring this empowering information by spending too much time and energy prescribing medications that can slow or dull the brain's ability to engage in its own healing. As a society we have become so conditioned to the notion that the patient is a passive participant, who only needs to be compliant with taking his or her pills every day, that we ignore our greatest resource: our brains.

One part of the brain with a proclivity for neurogenesis is the *hippocampus,* which is involved in activities related to learning and memory. Research shows that with the right stimulation, new neurons can be created in the hippocampus, even in older brains. You can think of the hippocampus as one of the farmer's crops: If planted in the right soil and right environment, and cared for appropriately, it will sprout, branch, and blossom with new neurons.

Research has shed some light on what type of "seeds," "soil," "water," and "air" the hippocampus favorably responds to. One is nutrients like proteins, which are the building blocks of cells. The body needs a plentiful supply of proteins in order to create new cells. And just as dangerous bugs and flies can kill crops, the hippocampus also needs a clean environment for growth. A diet abundant in copious amounts of antioxidants and inflammation-lowering foods provides the neurons with "clean air" and a good environment for neurogenesis.

Inflammation caused by poor eating habits and stress impedes neurogenesis. In fact, excessive cortisol created by stress can actually kill cells in the hippocampus. On the other hand, studies show that there is a strong positive relationship between exercise and neurogenesis. In fact, scientists like Gage have demonstrated that if you put a laboratory mouse on a running wheel and let it run, its hippocampus will spontaneously grow neurons even in the absence of new learning requirements. Researchers are not yet sure how exercise causes this to happen, but it seems that aerobic exercise works best. Even a twenty-minute walk has been shown to help.

Emotions also impact neurogenesis in the hippocampus. Depression, like stress, makes it harder for nerve cells to grow in that region of the brain, while positive mental activities have the opposite effect. Additionally, sleep deprivation retards neurogenesis, possibly by increasing the levels of stress hormones like cortisol.

Activities that challenge the mind stimulate it to produce cells in its learning centers. The brain doesn't change or develop when it's bored: It likes newness. Try to expose yourself to new things as much as possible. If your brain is—or is at risk of becoming—the equivalent of a "couch potato," look for ways to keep it active. Begin by keeping track of what you expose your brain to each day and how much of your day is spent actually moving as opposed to sitting or lying down. Gradually increase the number of "active minutes" during which your brain is engaged each day by participating in "brain exercises" such as

- Reading
- Playing games like chess
- Sudoku
- Playing a musical instrument
- Puzzles
- Taking a class

In case you didn't notice, mindless surfing of the Internet while your bottom is planted in a chair is not on our list.

Another positive mental activity that will help is *love*. Yes, that includes hand-holding, lip-smacking romance. Giving female mice a whiff of the scent of hunky male mice actually promotes hippocampus neurogenesis. Love and *nurturing* stimulate positive changes that promote learning. A loving and positive environment allows for growth and helps lower stress. I think it is pretty cool that the more kindness we spread to others, the healthier our minds become.

The Pain Matrix
The brain is made up of many different parts, including the hippocampus, brain stem, limbic system, and motor cortex. You might remember those colorful pictures from your high school biology textbook, the ones showing these various sections of the brain. None of those colored areas are responsible for handling pain—that is, for receiving pain information from various parts of the body, processing that data, and perhaps sending back a response (such as "pull your hand off of that hot stove," "stop putting weight on your sprained ankle," or "cry for help!"). That's because there is no single place in the brain where pain is handled, no single "pain center." Pain is a very complex phenomenon with several different components. It's a "package" of information with physical, emotional, and cognitive components that is dealt with simultaneously at various locations in the brain.

When a pain situation arises, the brain responds by producing a sensory component that tells us *what* we feel, an emotional component that tells us *how* we feel about it, as well as a cognitive component that determines what we *think* about the pain. Our evaluation of any pain experience, even a trivial one like bumping our knee against the side of a desk, takes place on all three levels simultaneously. For example:

Pain Situation: Stubbed Toe
Sensory component: Ouch!!!! Pain at level 8 on a scale of 1 to 10.
Emotional component: Irritation: Why did this happen to me?
Cognitive component: It's all right; it will stop hurting in a minute.

Pain Situation: Moderately Painful, Prolonged Chest Pain in Sixty-Year-Old Man
Sensory component: Pain at level 6 on a scale of 1 to 10.
Emotional component: Fear: Am I going to die?
Cognitive component: Stay calm and call 911.

Pain Situation: Chronic Back Pain Now in Second Year
Sensory component: Pain at level 3 on a scale of 1 to 10.
Emotional component: Fear, feeling of helplessness and hopelessness: When is this going to end? Will I ever be well? No one can help me!
Cognitive component: I need to ask my doctor to try different medications to help me feel better.

To these three components—sensory, emotional, and cognitive—we can add several more, which represent the brain's instructions to the body. For example

Pain Situation: Stubbed Toe
Sensory component: Ouch!!!! Pain at level 8 on a scale of 1 to 10.

Emotional component: Irritation: Why did this happen to me?

Cognitive component: It's all right; it will stop hurting in a minute.

Brain's instructions to body: Shift weight to undamaged foot, lift damaged foot, hold injured toe tightly with hands, make an ice pack.

Pain Situation: Moderately Painful, Prolonged Chest Pain in Sixty-Year-Old Man

Sensory component: Pain at level 6 on a scale of 1 to 10.

Emotional component: Fear: Am I going to die?

Cognitive component: Stay calm and call 911.

Brain's instructions to body: Trigger a fight-or-flight stress response (blood pressure rises, hands get clammy, breathing is rapid, and so on), clench fist next to chest.

Pain Situation: Chronic Back Pain Now in Second Year

Sensory component: Pain at level 3 on a scale of 1 to 10.

Emotional component: Fear, feeling of helplessness and hopelessness: When is this going to end? Will I ever be well? No one can help me!

Cognitive component: I need to ask my doctor to try different medications to help me feel better.

Brain's instructions to body: Produce more cortisol, increase blood pressure, store more fat, avoid moving as much as possible.

Taken all together, the sensory, emotional, and cognitive components plus the brain's instructions to the body make up the "*pain matrix,*" an intricate template that links all the places in the brain where pain is recognized and evaluated and responses to the pain are created.

Pinpointing the Action Areas

Exactly where in the brain does all this take place? Thanks to modern technology, we can "see" the brain in pain. One of the newest and most exciting ways to take pictures of the brain is called *functional magnetic resonance imaging* (fMRI). Regular MRI produces detailed pictures of the soft tissues, bones, and other internal structures. It works by sending out radio frequency signals to the body's atoms and using a computer to interpret the signals the atoms send back. MRIs are noninvasive and do not expose the patient to high levels of radiation.

fMRI takes this a step further. Even though the brain makes up only 2 percent of the body's weight, it receives 15 percent of the blood pumped by the heart, consumes 20 percent of the body's oxygen, and burns 25 percent of its glucose. Blood flow to the brain is continually and rapidly shunted to the parts that are most active and use up the most energy. The fMRI measures the way oxygen is taken up by different parts of the brain to determine which are active at any given time. fMRI allows us, for the first time ever, to determine exactly which parts of the brain are activated by a painful stimulus.

Seeing the Brain, Seeing the Power

Sean Mackey, MD, director of the Stanford Pain Clinic, is at the forefront of brain imaging research on pain. One of the most valuable lessons he has learned from his research is that seeing pictures of their brains has a powerful impact on chronic pain sufferers, for it allows them to see their pain in a tangible way. Finally they have something they can hold in their hands that helps explain what they are feeling and going through. It's like holding your own chest X-ray, the one that proves you have pneumonia. Mackey notes, "Pain is in the brain, and it's a private and personal experience unique to each person. There is lots of variability from person to person." No two fMRIs taken of subjects experiencing pain look exactly alike. Our distinct and unique experiences with pain come across in the diversity of our brains' pictures.

Some important health implications are starting to show up in Mackey's research. "Fear and anxiety seem to play a significant role in the experience of pain," he notes. He also says that there seem to be some general differences in the way brains of people experiencing pain look, compared to individuals who are asymptomatic. Some of these changes even suggest that chronic pain brains show signs of premature aging, although this still has not yet been proven. On the plus side, one of the things that excites him most about his research is watching the brain change in positive ways.

Mackey is conducting a number of brain imaging studies that are pushing his research into the frontiers of neuroscience. He is currently examining the links between depression and pain, identifying how love impacts pain perception, monitoring the brains of people with chronic pain when they are at rest, and tracking decision-making patterns in people with chronic pain. He is also beginning to do similar studies on parts of the spinal cord and eventually hopes to connect occurrences there with activity in the brain.

New research and developments like fMRI point to an exciting future in neuroscience. We've already learned that the brain is a complex organ with limitless potential to adapt, react, and grow in response to its environment. Each and every one of us has the power to control and guide these changes in positive directions. This means it is possible for you to learn to use your brain as a restorative tool and as a means of attaining good health and personal transformation.

Just Thinking about Pain . . .

Imagine looking at the brains of three different people: One has just received a painful stimulus such as an electric shock, the second is anticipating receiving a painful stimulus, while the third is watching a family member being shocked. If you follow their brains with fMRI, you can see that all three show increased activity in a part of the cortex known as the *anterior cingulate cortex* (ACC). However, none of the three show action in precisely the same spot of the ACC. Somehow the brain distinguishes between receiving a painful stimulus, waiting to receive one, and watching a loved one receive one and then reacts in a similar way but not exactly the same way to these three scenarios.

Why is this important? The ACC is involved with some very serious quality-of-life issues. Its functions include processing and evaluating information, initiating action or inaction, and handling emotional reactions. As a key part of the pain matrix, the ACC connects to several other areas of the brain and helps determine which actions we take, such as getting out of bed or going to the gym. When you're in pain, for example, the pain matrix shuts down the motivational parts of the brain. It also helps create an emotional response to your own pain—sad, hopeful, angry, nervous, and so on—and to the pain of others. Another section of the cortex, known as the *insula cortex,* is also involved in emotion; it influences activity in the brain associated with stress and contributes to some of the autonomic nervous system changes associated with stress that were discussed in chapter 6.

If You Know Where the Pain "Is" . . .

As soon as research scientists began mapping out the pain matrix, they also started to look for ways to use the matrix to combat pain. Was it possible to short-circuit pain by "turning off" certain parts of the matrix?

Studies with fMRI have demonstrated that the ACC is involved in the placebo effect, or the ability of a nonmedicinal substance—a so-called sugar pill— to quell pain. (Researchers have found that positive responses to placebos used to treat pain are in the 30 to 50 percent range. I bet you are surprised that the response rate is that high!) Specifically, these studies have shown changes in ACC activity when pain is relieved by a placebo. This does not mean you have to go out and buy a bottle of sugar pills to relieve your pain. It means you can begin to relieve your pain by trying to change your thoughts and/or beliefs about everything surrounding your pain.

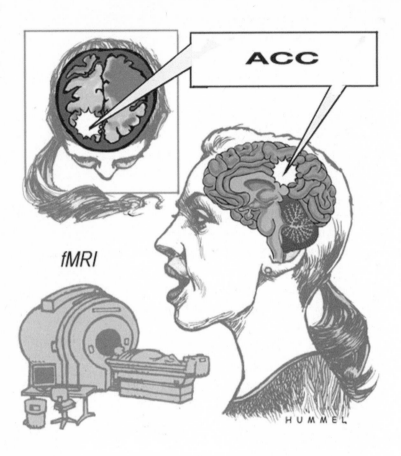

Researchers decided to test this theory by using distraction as a tool to help patients manage their pain. In these studies, certain parts of the brain, including the ACC, were found to send signals to other parts of the nervous system that quieted the pain message. Relaxation techniques triggered similar responses in the ACC and other parts of the brain.

What these studies tell us is that by tracking progress on fMRI images, patients can be taught how to control the activation of the ACC and other pain-related parts of the brain. This brings us to a historic point in pain management: We can teach chronic pain sufferers techniques that, when mastered, they can use to change their pain matrix for the better.

Literally "Thinking Down" Pain?

Research using fMRI to image the brain in real time is now being conducted. For some of these studies, patients are being taught to control brain activation in certain areas, such as the ACC, by watching changes on their real-time fMRI (rtfMRI). Early results suggest that they can actually lower their pain by focusing on controlling ACC activity. In other words, *control the brain, control the pain!*

Let's suppose, for example, you are the volunteer in the rtfMRI scanner, watching pictures of ACC activation. If we were to apply an uncomfortable amount of heat to your skin, you would see a corresponding increase in ACC activity, in real time. Now suppose we gave you a few tips on how to control this ACC activity—perhaps telling you to visualize yourself sipping a piña colada while lounging on a pristine tropical beach—then applied the heat again. Preliminary research suggests that you could utilize those tips to reduce ACC activity and experience less pain.

Let's take this concept a step further. Instead of using acute pain (heat), suppose we tested this out on people suffering from chronic pain. Again, preliminary studies suggest that chronic pain sufferers could lower their discomfort levels by learning how to reduce ACC activation. Mackey and other researchers are currently using rtfMRI to help patients learn to control their pain by reducing activity at specific parts of the brain.

Now that we know a little about how the different parts of the brain contribute to the experience of pain, doesn't it make sense to have that darn pain matrix work in our favor? For example, since we now know that this matrix houses a motivational center that tends to be inhibited by pain, shouldn't we consciously try to override it?

That means changing our actions, doing things we might otherwise avoid like taking a walk or going back to work. And if relaxation techniques can lower pain symptoms by altering the flow of information within the matrix, why not use these techniques every day? Since we know we can grow new neurons by stimulating our minds and exercising, why can't we remodel the matrix in such a way that pain would be permanently reduced? Exciting new research tells us that the mind should be the leader in the battle to overcome chronic pain and should not be negated by excess medication or misguided thoughts.

You might be thinking that this emphasis on the brain as a pain control tool overlooks the importance of physical ailments. Perhaps you have already said to yourself, "What good is a remodeled brain if I'm still stuck with the same old crooked back?" My response is that healing doesn't take place in just a specific part of the brain or in an isolated area of the body, like an arm. No, true healing only occurs when all parts of the whole participate—everything from the cortex and limbic system to muscles, nerves, and joints. And the brain has the power to make all of this a whole lot easier.

Next, we will learn how our spiritual side can help us harness our minds to make it a more powerful healing tool.

CHAPTER 8

Spirituality and Healing

Sometimes patients are startled when I tell them that they've already been given a powerful pain medicine. "Was it some injection or pill?" they ask. I explain that this "medicine" is and always has been within them, waiting to be put to use. We know that we come equipped with our own antibodies to fight infections, but where inside are we hiding this magical potion to treat pain? If you read the last chapter, then you have likely guessed that the answer lies within the mind, and I would say you are partially correct. As you will soon see, there is more to the mind than just the firing of a few pounds of neurons between your ears.

We can't locate the spirit inside the human body, but it's definitely there. It's the indefinable force that turns a bunch of atoms and molecules into you, a living being. It makes you a self-aware individual, yet connects you with all living creatures; gives you the capacity to feel emotional pain and experience great joy; makes you want to continue enjoying the best life has to offer; and offers you powerful tools to help make those wonderful dreams come true.

Unfortunately, chronic pain can act like a thick wall, separating you from your spirit. Sickness and suffering can cast a veil over your true self, and if that goes on for too long, you can lose touch with your *spirit*. When such a profound loss takes place, you need to reacquaint yourself with *you*—with your spirit—so that you can tap into the healing power of the brain.

A spiritual teacher I know who recently battled through chronic pain came to speak to a group of our patients. One of the patients later thanked me for helping him get reacquainted with his spiritual self; he thought he had lost it for good. He also mentioned that he was surprised that a medical person like me would endorse the importance and validity of spirituality in healing. This gentleman made me realize that as doctors we can often be guilty of coming across as too close-minded in our approach to healing.

This particular patient made one of the most dramatic recoveries our center has ever seen in only five short weeks of treatment. His left hand and arm had been crushed in a traumatic accident that occurred while he was at work, and he lost all functional use of it. He was able to completely and fully rehabilitate his left upper extremity to the point that you could no longer tell that it had been injured. In just over a month, his dystrophic limb looked as good as new! Sure, he worked extremely hard with his rehabilitation, but he also engaged his inner spiritual energy to create an amazing case study in healing.

Perhaps the best way to understand the healing power of the brain is to look at different "types" of brains, or more accurately, at the different ways in which the human brain can function and the effect it has on the body and health.

The Monk Brain

One of the more fascinating insights to emerge from fMRI scans is the ability to distinguish the brains of people who regularly engage in spiritual practice such as meditation from the brains of those who do not. Studies conducted on numerous monks, including the Dalai Lama, have shown that meditation can trigger positive changes on the brain that can be seen in fMRI scans. We learned earlier that specific areas of the brain deal with emotions. One of these areas is the *insula,* which communicates with other areas of the brain that control bodily functions such as heart rate. Because they are given training in meditation practices designed to develop love and compassion for others, monks show strong positive emotional changes in the insula and other related brain areas. The fMRI scans of monks who are well versed in meditation designed to develop love and compassion consistently differentiate themselves from scans of subjects with no such training.

These studies of monks' brains emphasize that what goes on in our brains, or more specifically *what we allow to go on in our brains,* influences our bodies as well as our minds. What you think really does matter. Your thoughts are the launching point of your journey. How can you be healthy if you don't think you can be healthy? If you believe that your body is doomed to function poorly, then you can't expect to be anything but disabled. As the Dalai Lama put it, "If you want others to be happy, practice compassion. If you want to be happy, practice compassion."

You can see the link between thoughts and happiness for yourself in little things every day. For example, holding a door open for a stranger requires a conscious decision to be polite and considerate. At the gym I've always noticed that when folks entering ahead of me hold the tall and heavy doors open for me, and I thank them, their smiles reveal the joy they experience from their kind act. On the other hand, people who let the doors shut in my face always look unhappy and focused elsewhere.

You may wonder, "If being healthy and happy is as easy as thinking that we can be either of these, why is it so hard to accomplish?" Again, I think the monks give us a clue: *They practice what they want to be good at.* They don't leave it to chance that they'll be kind and loving people. They meditate on focused thoughts, like bringing joy to someone else, over and over again. Practicing what you want to be good at is a time-honored technique, and it works. My poor seventh-grade son is trying to learn how to divide fractions right now. He won't be able to master the concepts without working through plenty of practice problems (I know my genes!). Similarly if you think about pain or anger all day long, you are in a sense practicing being in pain and anger. With time your practice will make you better at being in pain and anger and worse at feeling physically and emotionally good.

The Noisy Brain

Unfortunately, most of us do not quite have monk brains filled with thoughts of love and compassion. Instead our brains are crammed with noise and conflict as by-products of compulsive and incessant thinking. I'm not talking about clear, creative, and focused thinking, but rather what most of us do more of the time, which is let our minds wander aimlessly.

Letting our minds spin without focus or purpose is like letting a car engine race in neutral: The resulting roar is deafening but very unproductive. Most of us are unknowingly addicted to noisy thinking, which means we don't turn off our idle thoughts. We're addicted to this type of thinking and rarely clear the din from our heads.

What's the harm in letting the mind wander? One problem has to do with the brain's tendency to engage in repetitive thought patterns. You've seen this happen when a song gets stuck in your head. The song creates a constant background hum that never goes away. With this song playing incessantly in your head, driving you absolutely batty, it is much harder for your brain to focus on productive tasks.

Now suppose that instead of listening to the same song over and over again, your mind engages in a repetitive pattern of dysfunctional thoughts? Let's say, for example, that you hurt your back while lifting a heavy box at work. Your mind can replay negative thoughts about what happened for days, months, and even years! You may be correct in thinking that your boss forced you to lift a box that was too heavy, but telling yourself this every day for the next five or ten years won't serve you well. That is like playing the "My Boss Is a Jerk" song in your head all day every day, and expecting that it will eventually put you in a good mood. Obviously that won't happen. I know this sounds silly, but I see people torment themselves with this type of harmful internal chatter all the time, and they never find happiness until they learn to turn it off.

One of these folks was Thomas, a middle-aged man who played a certain scenario over and over in his head. Injured in a car accident several years earlier, which caused chronic neck and back pain, Thomas experienced frequent fits of rage and anger and seldom seemed happy. His mind was filled with thoughts about what the "miserable" insurance company and doctors should be doing for him but weren't. He constantly recounted the ways in which he was being shafted by the system. Even good things that happened to others became grist for his unhappiness mill. For example, if Thomas learned that another patient was given a new mattress by his insurance company, he became obsessed with the idea of getting one, too. He would stew about not having a new mattress all day long, and when his inner tension built to the bursting point, he would call and scream at his insurance representative or his lawyer. He resorted to trying to calm his nerves by drinking to excess, and his primary care doctor had to struggle to control Thomas's blood pressure.

I have known Thomas for years now, and every time he succeeds in getting something he feels entitled to, his mind becomes fixated on some other benefit he feels he should be given. His negative emotions, created by his thoughts, overwhelm his existence to the point where he is more often angry, depressed, or anxious than he is joyous. When he does experience bits of happiness—when he hears a funny joke or sees something interesting—he enjoys the moment, but it is always fleeting because his angry thoughts intervene and shove the happiness aside. And while he responds to humor, he never tells a joke or seeks it out. Thomas is trapped, and he can't see that he is his own captor.

One of the most important lessons I offer my patients is to help them see that every emotion is preceded by a thought. This is a basic principle of modern psychology. How you feel at any given moment is the product of whatever thoughts your mind has recently created. Leaving your emotions to the mercy of angry, repetitive "noise" will perpetuate negative emotions like rage, depression, and agitation and keep you from experiencing happiness and contentment.

The Emotional Brain

Emotions are the bridge that connects the mind to the body. In a simple sense you could say that the cortex thinks and processes thoughts, then passes that information on to areas such as the *insula,* where the emotions are created. In addition to converting thoughts into emotions, the *insula* communicates with parts of the brain that control what happens in the body. This flow that leads from thoughts to emotions to changes in the body is clearly shown in the fight-or-flight response, our hardwired reaction to danger.

As soon as we sense a threat, whether we hear, see, smell, or feel it, or simply think it's there, the brain lights up with action. This "danger" thought is converted into emotions, including fear, as well as a series of physical changes that prepare us to either fight for our lives or run away. As discussed earlier, the heart and lungs swing into high gear; blood is shifted away from the stomach and other nonessential areas and toward vital areas such as the muscles; the pupils dilate for better eyesight; the salivary glands, tear glands, stomach, and intestines are inhibited (put on hold); and the body is otherwise made ready for battle. All it takes is a sound, a sight, a smell, a touch, or even just a sense that something is wrong, and, well, have you ever seen those old war movies in which a ship that had been calmly steaming along is suddenly attacked? All at once the alarm starts blaring, men race up and down ladders, helmets and flack jackets are pulled on, doors are slammed and locked, ammunition is shoved into guns, and in no time at all the ship is ready for action.

The emotions associated with the fight-or-flight response—fear, terror—are easy to identify. But oddly enough, emotions can be hard to "*find.*" You would think they would have to be located in the mind, but we often "hide" them in our physical bodies in order to keep them quiet. Yet even when we do, the situation that created those harmful emotions may still be present in the mind, which means that new pain may be created to take the place of that which we have hidden.

I recently saw Sally, a seventy-year-old woman suffering from a long-standing spinal condition. Typically she sees me every few years for a special injection in her back that helps reduce her pain and allows her to play tennis, about which she is passionate. She came to see me so that I could repeat this procedure, only this time I learned that her beloved husband of half a century had suddenly passed away within the previous year. She had continued to remain very active in community activities after his death, and even took over some of his prior commitments. As a result she was now busier than she'd ever been.

Sally came back for a follow-up visit a few weeks after her procedure, stating that her back pain was worse than it had ever been. She didn't think the problem was caused by the injection, because she had never had a problem with it before. When I felt her lower back, I found a few very tight spots that were exquisitely painful to the touch. We sat and talked some more, and then she said, "You know, I have never had a chance to grieve for my husband's death." I believe she had unknowingly bottled up her sadness, storing it in her lower back, a place where she was already injured. The injection woke this terrible pain from its slumber, creating extremely painful spots that practically popped out at me.

The statue known as *The Thinker* is the most famous creation of one of history's most renowned sculptors, Auguste Rodin. *The Thinker* is depicted as a man in somber thought going through strong internal struggles. He is posed with his right knuckles under his chin, right elbow resting near the left knee, and sitting on a tree trunk in a crouched posture. His mind is agonizing over something, and his body is responding by contorting into this awkward position. He apparently has a lot of noise and thoughts in his head, and the more he thinks, the more he contorts his body. In this sense he is similar to people who suffer from chronic pain, who wrestle with their own internal struggles. They have lots of thoughts, and their outward appearance can change, reflecting their struggles. This statue has long been an icon of the intellectual mind.

I think this statue is an excellent illustration of the connection between thoughts, emotions, and the body. The head and face look down, suggesting a mind tormented by its own thoughts. The back is curved over the chest, and the shoulders are raised toward the ears, reminiscent of a creature in a defensive posture trying to protect itself during an attack. This is not a comfortable position—try holding it for a minute and you will see what I mean—and there is nothing in his body language that suggests his mind is open to anything other than the painful noise consuming his mind, body, and spirit. I think it is fair to say that his body is sharing the heaviness of his thoughts.

Sometimes you can find the crux of your self-destructive thoughts/negative emotions by tracing things backward from the body. Sally did it without even knowing it. Her "new" back pain, triggered by an injection that normally gave her relief, led her to recognize the emotion of grief, which had been bottled and hidden.

If chronic pain can cause a maelstrom of self-destructive thoughts and negative emotions, and if these connect the pain matrix in the brain to the body, then the result can be only one thing: more pain and more suffering! How do we break this vicious cycle?

The Mindful Brain

A mind liberated from idle chatter and repetitive negative thoughts is free to focus on helping the body to heal. You can achieve this liberation through meditation, prayer, and striving for stillness. I call the brain that achieves this the "mindful brain."

Developing a mindful brain requires focus, diligence, and plenty of practice. Remember: There are inherent, external barriers to this process. The noise inside our minds feeds directly off the cacophony that bombards us daily in the form of cell phones, computers, televisions, and the like. For most of us the external environment is a terrible distraction from mental clarity, which means we may need to make some disciplined lifestyle changes.

One important lesson that I have learned over the years is that dramatic cognitive and emotional changes can occur through movement and exercise. Remember: Emotions are the bridge between mind and body, and we know that the mind has the power to change the body. Conversely, the body has the power to influence the mind by changing emotions and thought patterns. It does this primarily through movement. The combined benefits of clearing the mind and moving the body are not just addictive; they are exponential. Part III of this book will introduce you to some different movement practices that have helped change the lives of hundreds of my patients.

I believe that putting the lid on dysfunctional, repetitive ideas is one important step toward conquering chronic pain. Another important step is to overcome internal conflict. My patients seem to suffer from an unconscious internal struggle between opposite forces that pull against each other. Until these conflicts are resolved, a person's life circumstances can stagnate and not move forward.

The Fearful Brain

The wicked stepmother in this chapter is fear. Fear starts to multiply and grow the minute pain first occurs. In the natural order of things, fear serves a protective function after an acute injury or some other form of stress. Every year kids at school fall off the monkey bars and break limbs. When they hit the ground, they may experience the severe pain caused by the sudden fracture of, say, a forearm. The immediate, inborn response is to cradle the injured arm to the chest with the good arm, protecting what has been injured from further damage.

Let's assume that most of these injuries are properly treated and heal within a few months. (Remember when you were that young and could heal, as good as new, so quickly?) Once the swelling and inflammation has gone down, kids usually start to regain full function of their limbs in a short time. Some may be a bit nervous about getting back up on the monkey bars, but most quickly get past that and resume their typical playful activities.

But if the pain persists even after an acute injury or fracture has healed, fear can become intertwined with the chronic pain. The fear of using a painful body part can persist; this is a reaction known as the *fear of reinjury*. In the case of our child injured at the playground, the fear of reinjury exists if the child is too scared to use the arm even after it has healed.

I have found that fear-based limitations are one of the biggest sources of physical impairment and emotional distress for patients with chronic pain. Fear can become an irrational bias preventing us from making appropriate and healthy decisions. The fear grows to the point where the body's operating systems start to shut down. I commonly see folks with injuries to an arm, for example, who struggle with pain *plus* significant limitations to what they can do with that arm. They may not be able to comb their hair or dress themselves with that arm, for example. In some cases they can't move the arm at all. For example, the shoulder socket can get rigid and stuck following a rotator cuff tear. If the tear is surgically repaired, but the shoulder remains frozen and resistant to movement, then fear might be contributing to the problem. Unfortunately, as you will learn in the next chapter, the longer the shoulder stays frozen, the more it will hurt and the weaker the arm will become.

I also see people who are worried that doing something might cause them to become seriously injured again. They fear, for example, "If I exercise, I could injure myself further." And believe it or not, some actually have a fear of getting better. They are accustomed to their role as the sick one—and perhaps accustomed to some of the benefits that come with it, such as extra attention from friends and family. Without realizing what is happening, they unconsciously allow their fear of letting go of the extra attention block out thoughts of getting better.

Does that mean that the fear of reinjury is all in your head? Certainly not. It is born out of real injuries and real pain. Fear taking hold within the mind is what freezes the body, preventing it from functioning. The end result is less activity, fulfillment, and joy. The fear takes the place of movement and achievement in life, making people prisoners of its whims and wishes.

The Faith Brain: The Antidote to Fear

Creating a mindful brain for yourself can be a powerful step toward regaining control, but it may not be enough in the face of over-whelming fear. As far as I'm concerned, fear is an emotional "germ" that needs to be cleansed or it will destroy the spirit. That's why the next step is to add faith—the true antidote to fear: faith that things can and will get better, faith that *you* can and will get better. Fear cannot live when faith is present.

When I see patients who have been even mildly infected with fear, I like to prescribe a large dose of faith. I wish I could simply hand them a bottle of "faith pills" or give them a "faith injection," but of course that's impossible. So instead, I encourage them to start thinking "I can," as in "I *can* use my arm again," "I *can* regain control of my life," "I *can* change my lifestyle for the better," "I *can* improve my relationships," "I *can* let go of my anger," "I *can* do more for myself than I am doing now," and "I *can* see a brighter future."

Deliberately filling your mind with "I can" thoughts turns the brain away from fear and noise, helping you create a "monk brain" that constantly thinks about the hopeful future, as well as a mindful brain, which silences the "can't" and other chatter and replaces them with positive, hopeful thoughts. The faith brain has all the positive attributes of these two brains, plus more, because focusing on "I can" is a powerful healer.

The actions that this creates can boost confidence and create a foundation from which to build. Being able to lift a frozen shoulder just a tad higher, for example, adds positive reinforcement to a person's faith that her arm will get better. It tells her that by next week, if she keeps at it, she probably will be able to raise it yet even higher. Faith can grow one step or one inch at a time, along with each accomplishment. Here are examples of changes in thought patterns that can help build a faith brain:

Instead of saying	Think
This pain is terrible!	I *can* conquer this pain.
Why bother? I'll never get better.	I *can* work through this therapy and I *can* get better.
Why did this happen me?	I *can* be healthy and whole again.
My family is driving me crazy over my pain.	I *can* communicate with them and improve our relationships.
Why can't those idiot doctors fix this?!	I *can* be an active part of my recovery.
I have so far to go, there's no point even trying.	I *can* take a little step forward today.
No one understands what I'm going through.	I *can* communicate what I need to, without coming across as a complainer.
I will never be the way I used to be, physically.	I *can* make great strides forward.
I'll never be the way I was.	I *can* live a happy and productive life, despite some physical limitations.

I don't want to make it sound like all you have to do is click your heels together three times, think happy thoughts, and everything will be perfect. It's not that easy. But it's not that hard, either. Keep thinking "I can," and look for ways to make every thought and every utterance an "I can" one. Even if you don't believe it at first, just say it. Eventually all of those "I can" thoughts and utterances will be written into the book of your mind, and each new "I can" thought and utterance will become easier—and easier and easier—until "I can" thinking is second nature to you.

The Vivaldi Brain

If there is one constant in nature, it is that there are four seasons that will continue to repeat themselves indefinitely. All around us, living creatures deal with these cycles. The leaves of the trees wither and fall every autumn. The trees come back to life each spring, when the leaves and blossoms return. This is the natural order of the universe. Life goes through cycles. Our challenge is to be like the trees, to take injuries and painful challenges (winter) and allow them to let us grow and bloom into more vibrant living creatures (spring). Being stuck seems to defy a basic law of the universe, which is that winter is always followed by spring. Each struggle is a potential door to growth and development if we are bold enough to walk through.

The Vivaldi brain lives in the moment and addresses what needs to be done at that particular time, whether it is a big challenge or something quite joyous. It learns the lessons of the harsh winter, then applies what it has learned to create a bright and bountiful spring. It never judges the flow of the seasons; instead it accepts them all. Some patients ask me every week what I think their future will be like: "Will things eventually go away?" I tell them that while I don't possess a crystal ball, I do think that they need to work on managing the pain that they have at that particular moment and take tomorrow as it comes.

In chapter 11, we will focus more closely on the simple act of breathing. Religious scholars have pointed out that the Hebrew word for spirit is *ruah,* which literally means "breath, air, or wind." Their conception of life and spirit is intricately connected to the breath. When we are born, the first thing we do is take a breath, and when we die, it is the final act we perform.

Ruah brings us to an important point about spirituality that dictionaries can't define. Breathing is the act of moving air into and out of our bodies. The wind blows from place to place. Our spirits are not purely self-contained. Thanks to the wind, they move and interact with our environment, including with the people around us. Our spirit impacts the lives of our family members, our loved ones, our coworkers, and others—and theirs impact ours as well. We've all heard how a special person can light up a room simply by entering it. Just as internal factors like thoughts and emotions impact the spirit we create, so too do external factors of our environment.

Patients and colleagues often ask me how I'm able to work all day every day with people who are in pain. I was recently talking with a patient who is a minister, when I finally figured out the true answer. He told me that he sometimes talks in his sermons about how I comforted him during dark times. I now realize that I feed off of the positive energy given out by people like him who make changes and become well, inside and out. This flow of energy charges me to do the same for the next person. But I can't continue without the help of those who I have already worked with. He breathes out his *ruah,* and I breathe it in, making it a part of my *ruah,* which I then breathe out to the next person.

Coming Back to Life

Chronic pain can wreak havoc on the body. And it can do the same to the mind by creating dysfunctional noises and tipping the scales away from faith and toward fear, leaving us with heavy emotions that blanket our true spirits. It is the good thoughts we create during times of stress and crisis that can serve as the glue that holds our body, mind, and spirit together. Just as the darkness of night yields to the brightness of the sun, every tragedy and struggle will give way to enlightenment and incredible gifts— joy, love, and serenity—if we let it.

Recall the story of Moses. One day he was a fugitive shepherd wandering the desert with his flock, and the next he was parting the Red Sea while rescuing a whole nation of people. What led to this remarkable transformation? God called him to action by speaking to him through a burning bush, and Moses listened, even though he didn't think he was a worthy choice. Your pain, illness, or suffering may be your burning bush, telling you what you can accomplish. The best medicine is to reconnect with your spirit and let it infuse you once again with the joy of living.

What Kind of Brain Do You Want?

I suggest you make a list of ideas you cling to about your pain, your health, and your life. Try to identify negative thoughts that you carry as part of your background chatter. This should include thoughts about other people and places, as well as self-directed opinions. Can you think of any fears you harbor that can hold you back? Next to each item on your list, try to write an alternative thought that would help you move in a more positive direction. Once you complete each chapter in Part III, get out your list and take a few moments to add new ideas that come to mind based on what you have read. Keep this sheet of paper in a safe place and refer back to it periodically, until you believe that you have made lasting changes.

Now it's time to move on and learn more about how the fear of reinjury can make pain even worse.

CHAPTER 9

Move It or Lose It: Why Inactivity Hurts

One of the most significant contributors to chronic pain is also one of the biggest health problems in our modern society: inactivity. I guess we can define this paradoxically as "the action of no action," which means this chapter is about what happens when nothing happens.

It's plain and simple: Inactivity hurts. A surefire way to make chronic pain worse is to avoid moving what already hurts. Inactivity can also set the stage for the development of a frightening number of new problems, ranging from muscle pain to fatal heart attacks. Indeed, there is a very close association between inactivity and the most prominent diseases of our time, including coronary artery disease, diabetes, and degenerative arthritis. Inactivity is a huge contributor to obesity, which is now at an epidemic level in the United States. Our battle with the bulge, in turn, directly contributes to other common problems, like heart disease, back pain, and diabetes. For example, the incidence of diabetes has risen so much that it, too, has become an epidemic. Some experts believe that overall life expectancy is now starting to decline due to the preponderance of overweight people. In 2005, the National Institutes of Health reported, "Over the next few decades, life expectancy for the average American could decline by as much as 5 years unless aggressive efforts are made to slow rising rates of obesity."[7]

And even if it doesn't kill us, obesity can make our lives more difficult in many ways. For example, excessive body weight puts more stress on weight-bearing joints like hips and knees, causing them to degenerate faster than normal. This means that moving too little can actually wear your body parts out more quickly!

---

7   "Obesity Threatens to Cut U.S. Life Expectancy, New Analysis Suggests." NIH News, National Institutes of Health, U.S. Department of Health and Human Services, March 16, 2005. Accessible at www.nih.gov/news/pr/mar2005/nia-16.htm.

You Practically Have to Make an Appointment to Move

It used to be very easy to move about, walk, engage your muscles in activity, lift or pull things, move items from here to there, and otherwise be active. In fact, you could not avoid doing so unless you were bedridden. Consider the simple act of sending a message to a distant friend. Many years ago we would have had to write a letter by hand, then walk or ride a horse to a post office to mail it. Twenty years ago we would have written the letter by hand, then stood up, walked to the front door, and placed it in the mailbox. Ten years ago we would have typed the letter and then maybe walked to the fax machine to send the letter. Now millions of Americans simply sit at their desks and send messages, pictures, and full documents by e-mail with just a few clicks of their fingers, practically eliminating the need to move at all. Don't get me wrong—this new technology is great, but relatively few muscles and almost no calories are burned sending e-mails.

Similarly, a century ago taking a trip might have required saddling a horse or hitching a wagon. Today it's as easy as putting a key into the ignition or swiping a pass through the scanner at a subway turnstile. One hundred years ago making dinner was a complex operation. You might have had to slaughter and dress a cow to get a steak or maybe walk a mile to the butcher shop (there were no home freezers to store your meat). You might have had to go to the garden and pick the broccoli, carrots, or other vegetables you had planted, then wash and chop them. And before you could cook the steak and vegetables, you would have had to chop your own wood, haul it into the kitchen, and set it in the hearth. Finally you would have had to make and tend to the fire and haul heavy metal pots and pans back and forth. Making a simple dinner could be exhausting! And we're not even talking about cleaning up afterward. Today it's easy to whip up a dinner of steak and mixed vegetables. You take the steak out of the freezer and pop it into the microwave, open a can of vegetables, and heat them in a pot on the stove.

For most of us the modern lifestyle is really a "sitstyle," with little physical effort required to get through the day. The problem is even more serious for suburbanites, who spend an inordinate amount of their time barely moving at all. Folks who live in metropolitan areas usually walk from their homes to public transit stops or, if the destination is not too far away, walk all the way. They also typically climb stairs every day and often carry groceries or other purchases from the stores to their homes. Suburbanites, on the other hand, generally get into their cars in their garages and drive themselves to work, the shopping center, and other destinations. They park the car as close to the entrance as possible, so they don't have to walk much. Thus the process of traveling several miles from home may burn very little in the way of "people energy." Purchases are transported home by car, not carried by hand. With cell phones, iPods, game consoles, and other computer gear, it's no longer necessary to seek out friends, go to the clubhouse, or go to the local gathering spot to be entertained. We don't even have to walk out to the backyard and shout something over the fence to a neighbor; we can have our Blackberry notify his. Suburb dwellers typically burn less energy than their urban counterparts, so it's no surprise that suburban living is associated with a greater risk of health problems, including obesity and depression.

Suburban Living Can Also Be Bad for Your Brain

Brains that are regularly stimulated and exposed to new things are less likely to develop forms of dementia than less-engaged brains. This can be a problem for suburbanites, who, living far from the city or community center, often find it difficult to attend meetings and concerts, meet with friends, or simply connect with others. As a result they may have less to do with other people, the community, and nature, while spending more time engaging in sedentary activities like sitting on the couch and watching television. TV can be entertaining, but it rarely "exercises" the mind.

Certain people still have to move quite a bit at work, but most of us can get by with doing very little every day.

Up to Our Ears in Shoulders

Our modern sitstyle has triggered a large number of pain problems related to the fact that we move so little. Twenty years ago few people had personal computers at home, and most probably didn't own cell phones. Today, however, many jobs require almost continuous work at computer workstations. This means keyboarding, using a mouse, and sitting in a fixed position for hours on end. And, after a full day of keyboarding and mouse moving at work, folks seem to spend more and more of their leisure time surfing the Internet and playing computer games.

What does all this hunching over computers do to our bodies? The next time you have a chance, observe a group of people working at computer-based workstations. Watch them for about an hour to get a good idea of how much—or little—they move. How often do they shift their necks and lower backs? Do they keep their elbows flexed the whole time? Are their shoulders shrugged up close to their ears? How much weight-bearing activity, like standing or walking, occurs? You will notice that there isn't a lot of movement going on in their joints and that their biggest muscles, those in their legs and back, are used infrequently.

When a body works in a semifixed position for endless periods of time, it starts to adapt by overengaging certain muscles needed to hold things in place, and turning off other muscles not directly related to the task. Most of us have a tendency to overactivate our upper trapezius muscles (which run down the back of the neck, shoulders, and upper back) when we do fine-motor activities with our hands because it helps hold our fingers, hands, wrists, and forearms up while we work. If you take your hand, place it at the base of your neck and slide it down sideways to the horizontal plane topping your shoulder, it will be resting on your trapezius. Pinch the muscle and see how it feels. Does it seem knotted up? This muscle often gets overstimulated not only by repetitive use of the hands, but by emotional stress, as well.

At the same time the trapezius is tightening, other muscles around the shoulder blades get turned off and stop working. These muscles are important for stabilizing the shoulder joints, and normally they work in concert with the trapezuis. But with the trapezius "on" so often and the other muscles "off," the balance tips and will lead to postural changes. The shoulders and neck start to stiffen and lose function.

The human body was designed for movement, not stagnation. We used to move, move, move all day long. Now we typically sit still for prolonged periods at work, take a sedentary trip home, perform more sedentary activities in the evening, and then lie down in bed all night. We overuse some muscles while ignoring others. The more we do this to our bodies, the more likely they will start to hurt. There was a time where most injuries were caused by sports or industrial accidents. While these types of injuries still occur, I now see lots of pain problems caused by just the opposite—inactivity.

Frozen in Fear

Not only does our modern sitstyle practically force us to be physically immobile much of the day, many of us are literally afraid to move, even when we have the opportunity. This phenomenon occurs when people who already hurt feel they can't possibly exercise because it will hurt even more. This is the fear of reinjury, or the fear avoidance model. For example, research has shown that people who tear their anterior cruciate ligament (ACL)—the knee injury that left me pantless—and who fear reinjury are more likely to avoid playing their sport again.

Experience has taught me that fear of movement is one of the biggest obstacles to winning the battle against pain. Just as the fear of reinjury can cause athletes to avoid returning to certain activities after an injury, it appears to have a similar effect on a large proportion of my patients with chronic pain. They may have slipped on ice

and injured a tailbone or injured themselves while lifting or trans-
ferring a loved one, but now they avoid doing anything that might
cause a recurrence. This is natural: When we experience lots of pain,
we respond by guarding and protecting our bodies. It is as if we
are trying to curl up in a protective shell and hide until the danger
passes. Venturing out of this shell leaves us feeling exposed to the
risks of further injury and more discomfort.

Protecting an acutely injured part of the body is a normal and
useful response that helps prevent further damage until the injury
can heal. For example, if you sprain your ankle, it gets swollen,
inflamed, and painful. The more you try to stand on it, the more it
hurts. This pain and your desire to avoid it keep you off of the ankle
until it has a chance to heal. Once the ankle has healed, it no longer
hurts to walk on it.

A chronic pain situation is a different matter, however. Typically, by the time the pain has become chronic, the acute injury
has already healed, so it no longer needs to be protected. Once a
sprained ankle has healed, for example, staying off of the ankle actually makes it worse. In order for the muscles around the leg and foot
to get strong again, they need to be worked. The less they are used,
the more they will atrophy. If the joint isn't flexed and straightened, it will remain stiff. It will then begin to freeze and scarring
will develop, which will keep it from moving the way it did before.
Pretty soon the leg is limping, which triggers low back pain. And if
the back is overprotected, it too will freeze, throwing the body out
of alignment and triggering pain somewhere else.

Another fear is that moving or using the damaged area will
cause further damage. If the ankle hurts, the mind might be fooled
into thinking that walking on it will damage it, even though the
sprain occurred six months earlier. Did I say "fooled"? Yes, chronic
pain can con us into believing things about ourselves and our bodies
that may not be true.

Some folks dwell on their physical symptoms to the point
where they believe they are continually in harm's way. Recall from

chapter 2 that a doctor's words can trigger such anxiety. A patient may become terrified of becoming paralyzed, for example, even though the odds of that happening are usually rather remote. Other patients may tend to catastrophize, or believe things are worse than they really are. These folks are at a greater risk of avoiding movement out of fear.

No matter what the reasons for it, inactivity is unhealthy. It causes us to develop rigid, poorly functioning muscles, which hurt once we try to use them again. The less active we are, the weaker and more deconditioned our muscles become. Our joints depend on properly functioning muscle groups for support, so we also run the risk of wearing out our joints prematurely if we do not maintain adequate muscle strength. This eventually leads to painful arthritis. Our spine also benefits from the active support of key muscle groups to help with posture and stability so we don't slouch or put excess pressure on our joints in order to remain upright. What's more, avoiding movement eventually leads us down a path to serious health risks such as obesity, osteoporosis, diabetes, and heart attack. And obesity continues the vicious cycle by putting added stress on important joints like the knees and hips, leading to inflammation and degeneration of the supporting cartilage, and of course, lots of pain.

Once you've finished reading this chapter, take a few moments to consider your painful areas, how you think of them, and how you use (or don't use) them. Is it time to reevaluate your thoughts and change your beliefs about your situation? Changing some of your ideas and behaviors could be the first step toward creating a new and vibrant you.

The Terrible Toll of Not Toiling

Many studies have shown that inactivity and obesity are risk factors for some of the major diseases of our day. Here's a sampling of the studies:

- **Heart disease in men.** From the *Journal of the American Medical Association:* "Total physical activity, running, weight training, and walking were each associated with reduced CHD risk."[8] CHD stands for coronary heart disease, a major killer. This study followed over 44,000 men for over a decade to find that moving was good medicine for the heart.

- **Stroke in women.** From the *Journal of the American Medical Association:* "Physical activity including moderate-intensity exercise such as walking, is associated with a substantial reduction in risk of total and ischemic stroke in a dose-response manner."[9] There are two types of stroke: ischemic and hemorrhagic. With an ischemic stroke the blood flow to a part of the brain is cut and brain neurons die—this is like a heart attack. With a hemorrhagic stroke, a blood vessel in the brain "breaks" and blood floods into the brain "drowning" neurons. This study found that exercise reduces the risk of both types of stroke added together, as well as ischemic stroke by itself. And it did so in a dose-response manner, which means that more exercise provided more benefit, while less exercise provided less benefit.

- **Type II diabetes.** From *Diabetes Care:* Participating "in physical activities of moderate intensity such as brisk walking can substantially reduce the risk of type 2 diabetes."[10] To arrive at this conclusion, the researchers looked at ten different studies of physical activity and type 2 diabetes involving over 300,000 people. They found that regularly participating in moderately intense physical activity reduced the risk of developing type 2 diabetes by some 30 percent.

---

8 Tanasecu, M., Leitzmann. M.F., Rimm, E.B., et al. "Exercise type and intensity in relationship to coronary heart disease in men." *JAMA* 2002; 288(10):1994–2000.

9 Hu, F.B., Stampfer, M.J., Colditz, G.A., et al. "Physical activity and risk of stroke in women." *JAMA* 2000; 283(12):2961–2967.

10 Jeon, C.Y., Kokken, R.P., Hu, F.B., van Dam, R.M. "Physical activity of moderate intensity and risk of type 2 diabetes: a systematic review." *Diabetes Care* 2007; 30(3):744–752.

- **Rectal cancer.** From the *International Journal of Cancer:* "Physical inactivity, high energy intake and obesity are associated with the risk of rectal cancer, and there is a probable synergic effect among the 3 risk factors."[11]

- **Breast cancer in men.** From the *Journal of the National Cancer Institute:* "Obesity was positively related . . . and physical activity inversely related . . . " to the risk of developing breast cancer in men in this study.[12] "Positively related" means that as obesity increased, so did the risk of developing the cancer. "Inversely related" means there was an opposite association: As exercise levels *increased,* cancer risk *decreased.* This study found that keeping the weight down and the exercise level up was protective.

- **Endometrial and breast cancer.** From *Cancer:* The authors of this study began by noting that "convincing epidemiologic evidence links excess body mass to increased risk of endometrial and postmenopausal breast cancers. . ."[13] "Epidemiologic evidence" is the kind you derive when you look at large populations and compare, in this case, certain aspects of their lifestyle habits to their health.

- **Colorectal cancer.** From *Cancer Epidemiology, Biomarkers and Prevention:* "Obesity has a direct and independent relationship with colorectal cancer."[14] For this meta-analysis or "marriage of studies," the researchers used statistical means to combine the results of thirty-one different studies. Specifically, they found that for every 2-kilogram increase in BMI (see pages 121–123 for more information), the risk of developing colorectal

---

11 Mao, Y., Pan, S., Wan, S., Johnson, K. "Physical inactivity, energy intake, obesity and the risk of rectal cancer in Canada." *Int. J. Cancer* 2003; 105(6):831–837.

12 Brinton, L.A., Richesso, D.A., Gierach, G.L., et al. "Prospective evaluation of risk factors for male breast cancer." *J. Nat'l. Cancer Inst.* 2008; 100(20):1477-81.

13 Leitzmann, M.F., Koebnick, C., Danforth, K.N., et al. "Body mass index and risk of ovarian cancer." *Cancer* 2009; 115(4):812-822.

14 Moghaddam, A.A., Woodward, M., Huxley, R. "Obesity and risk of colorectal cancer: a meta-analysis of 31 studies with 70,000 events." *Cancer Epidemiol Biomarkers Prev.* 2007; 16(2):2533-47.

cancer rose by 7 percent, and for every 2-centimeter (about 0.8 inch) increase in waist circumference, the risk rose by 4 percent.

I could go on and on with the studies, but the point is clear: Both lack of exercise and obesity are linked to debilitating and deadly diseases.

How Much Is Too Much?

Simply stepping on a scale and seeing how much you weigh is not the best way to determine whether your weight is harming your health. That's because a "healthy weight" for one person may be a threatening number of pounds for another, even if they are about the same height. Compare two women: One is 5'8" and weighs 185 pounds, with most of her excess weight in her belly. The other, standing just as tall and tipping the scales at the same 185 pounds, carries most her extra weight in her thighs and buttocks. The first woman is what we call an "apple," round in the middle and slimmer on top and bottom, while the second is a "pear," slimmer up above and rounder down below. This is more than a matter of aesthetics, for fat carried around the belly tends to be more metabolically active and hence more dangerous than fat stored in the thighs and buttocks.

There are a few simple measurement tools you can use to gauge whether or not you are overweight besides simply weighing yourself.

Measurement Tool #1: BMI
A common tool for measuring the risk of disease and mortality linked to body composition is known as the body mass index, or BMI. Calculating BMI requires you to plug your weight and height into this rather complicated formula:

BMI = weight (in pounds) x 703/ height (in inches)

If you prefer to skip the calculation, you can use the Centers for Disease Control and Prevention's online BMI calculator found at www.cdc.gov/nccdphp/dnpa/healthyweight/assessing/bmi/adult_BMI/english_bmi_calculator/bmi_calculator.htm. Just type in your height and weight, click on "Calculate," and the computer figures it out for you.

What should your BMI be? The risk for men goes up when BMI exceeds 25.3, and for women it goes up when the value exceeds 24.3.

Measurement Tool #2: Waist-to-Hip Ratio
As mentioned, fat stored in the abdominal area—that is, wrapped around the waist—has been shown to be more harmful than fat stores in other areas of the body. Having more weight around your waist than around your hip area increases the risk of developing heart disease and diabetes.

To figure your waist-to-hip ratio, use a tape measure to measure your hip circumference (all the way around your hips at the widest part) and then your waist (just above the upper hip bone). Divide the waist circumference by your hip circumference to get your ratio. For example:
If your hip is 36 inches and your waist is 24 inches, your ratio is 0.67.
If your hip is 42 inches and your waist is 38 inches, your ratio is 0.90.
If your hip is 46 inches and your waist is 40 inches, your ratio is 0.87.

What is a healthy ratio? For men it should be below 0.94, and for women it should be below 0.82. Higher figures suggest danger.

Which Measurement Should You Use?
Neither BMI nor waist-to-hip ratio is a perfect predictor of health

or disease, so it's best to use both. If your results on either test are in the danger zone, speak to your doctor about your diet and exercise regimens.

Great News!

There is some great news amid all this discussion of inactivity, weight, and disease: Keeping your weight under control will help reduce your risk of developing many of the major diseases of our time. It may play a role in keeping your pain under control, too. The fear of reinjury is a very beatable foe. Once you overcome the fear, you will be amazed at what you can do. With the right education, insight into your limitations, and an understanding of where your unneeded fears reside, you can work past limitations and barriers. People who are able to do this often enjoy tremendous physical gains. Those who were once able to lift and carry only a pound may find they can soon carry twenty pounds. Those who could only tolerate five minutes of walking on a treadmill may soon go twenty minutes on an incline. Their bodies become much stronger, rapidly. Their general outlook on life and feeling of control improves, too.

It *is* doable. I've seen it happen many times, and I've seen people completely turn their lives around once they start to "move it" again.

Now that you've learned valuable truths and sharpened your mind for success, it's time to dare yourself to dive headfirst into the learning process and begin the extreme makeover that will help you put your pain in its place!

PART III:

DARE

CHAPTER 10

Seven Steps to an Extreme Makeover

What are the key traits of highly successful chronic pain sufferers? In other words, what are the differences between those who effectively overcome chronic pain and those who do not? Having worked with thousands of patients, I have had an opportunity to witness firsthand both positive and negative outcomes, many times over. Through my observation and research, I have found the key ingredients for a chronic pain makeover and I'm going to share them with you here. After all, everywhere you turn, from television shows to print, there is a wealth of advice devoted to helping you radically improve your appearance. If experts can teach you how to have great hair and look sexier, then it's high time you got some advice on how to transform the way you feel, too!

Let's suppose that two forty-five-year-old women with severe low back pain come to my center with similar problems. They both were once very active and enjoyed recreational activities like hiking and tennis, but now they are in too much pain to do those sports. Both women have families, but they find themselves snapping at their kids and spouses in ways they never did before the pain began. The fact that they struggle to complete chores makes them feel less needed and more depressed; this sadness often brings them to tears. Each is taking a combination of potent painkillers and antidepressants, but both note that the pain seems to get worse and worse.

Now let's pull out a crystal ball and see where our two patients will be a year from now. One woman will be about the same. Even though she tried various treatments over the last year, her back still hurts a lot, so she still spends a lot of time lying down. She continues to take strong pain medications and feels emotionally low. Her relationship with her husband is more strained than ever, and the two struggle to communicate with each other.

Things look considerably brighter for our other patient. She is much more active and cheerful. When friends ask her about her back, she lets them know that she still feels some discomfort, but it will no longer keep her from their weekly get-togethers. She spends a few hours every day doing the things that she learned to take better care of her back, but this leaves her with plenty of quality time for her kids and husband.

Why the discrepancy between the two women? My guess is that our first patient acquired few, if any, of the healthful habits I'll be describing in this chapter. Experience dictates, however, that the second patient brought many of these steps into her daily life and kept them there.

Let's not forget one of the valuable lessons of the first two parts of this book. Contact time, or more to the point, how *you* use your time, is a critical factor. Granted, using your contact time to your best advantage is no small challenge; it requires a supreme, unwavering effort. Consider Lance Armstrong. Is he not a naturally gifted physical specimen ideally suited for bike racing? Well, yes, but so are a lot of other creatures inhabiting our planet, whether they pedal or not. What set Armstrong apart from the pack during his unprecedented string of seven *Tour de France* victories was that he worked harder. Absolutely committed to success, he never let anyone outtrain him. Armstrong proves that success doesn't just *happen.* Even exceptionally talented people can't just show up for a race expecting to win. They know they must train harder than their competition. The same applies if you want to be victorious over chronic pain: You must outwork it to take charge.

The following seven steps will help you create a training regimen to win the battle against chronic pain. Don't worry about delving into the details of each step right now; what follows is just a quick overview. I'll spend more time in the chapters that follow talking about these and other helpful things you can do to overcome your pain. And don't worry about tackling the parts in order; that's not necessary. You don't have to master one before moving on to the next. Try them all. Some will feel comfortable right away; others will take more time. Don't worry about that; just keep moving ahead.

Step One: Use Your Breath

Learning how to use your breath is a fundamental step toward gaining control of your health. Your breath is the root from which all your branches will sprout. Mastering the breath can help you

- Stretch tight muscles
- Strengthen parts of the body overprotected by the fear of pain
- Boost your energy and endurance
- Manage pain flare-ups
- Reduce stress
- Clear your mind of negative chatter
- Get a better night's sleep

Step Two: Create a Healing Mind

Chapters 7 and 8 taught us that the mind is a powerful tool for improving health and wellness. If we aren't careful, we can easily allow dysfunctional thoughts to take root in our minds. Acting through the mind/body connection, harmful thoughts throw us off track. They create negative emotions that "speak" to our bodies, setting in motion biochemical and physiological changes that can worsen our pain and cause our physical bodies to shut down. New research now shows that if we can control our brain, we can control our pain. In order to help you accomplish this, upcoming chapters will focus on

- Breathing and meditative exercises to reduce stress, cleanse negative thoughts and emotions, and replace them with healing alternatives such as gratitude and appreciation
- Learning the value of acceptance, not as a path to defeat but as a means of improving emotional well-being

- Becoming acquainted with the ways in which the creative side of your brain can process bottled-up negative emotions that need to be released
- Recognizing how addiction to prescription pills, alcohol, and drugs can control your decision making and block helpful thoughts
- Understanding how hard-to-see dependencies, such as emotional addictions to anger or fear, can be equally dangerous

Step Three: Connect

Some of my happiest patients are those whom I consider to be the most "connected." Connections are the bonds we form with the world around us. For example, I see many patients who were injured at work and need to take a leave of absence while they seek treatment. This time off may be necessary, but it can also be harmful in that it allows the work connection to weaken. A work connection can provide valuable intangibles to life, including social bonds and a feeling of purpose. Breaking this bond can send many people into a tailspin. But the ones who later establish new connections, either by returning to work or finding something that replaces work, like volunteering, seem to manage their pain much better.

Many people react to their chronic pain experience by retreating from more than just work. They may cut down on or avoid social contacts, like visiting with friends or going to church. *But each interaction you miss out on removes a connection from your life.* As connections become fewer and fewer, the world around you becomes smaller and smaller. Preserving your connections, or creating new ones, significantly improves the quality of your life.

As you branch out, look to make healthy bonds. Seek out friends who like to take walks or exercise. Get involved in pursuits where you can share your love and kindness with others. This will bring more healing into your life than you can ever imagine.

The information contained in the upcoming chapters on exercise, home life, healthy aging, facing addiction, and gaining acceptance will help you eliminate the physical and emotional barriers to your connections.

Step Four: Ingest Quality

Our bodies are totally dependent on the air we breathe and the nutrients we eat to run properly. But each and every day we expose our bodies to chemicals from the food we consume and the medications we take. We often lose sight of the fact that our health hinges on every breath and swallow that takes place.

View your body as a temple and cherish everything you put into it. Consider carefully what medications you will expose it to. To keep it in tip-top shape, you must be committed to ingesting only quality substances. Whenever possible, adhere to the principles of the Anti-Inflammatory Diet discussed in chapter 15. Chapters 14 and 21 will help you make decisions about your long-term medication goals.

Step Five: Add Balance

There are only so many hours in a day, and as you will see, you need to spend a third of it sleeping. If you want to take charge of your pain, you need to strike the right balance in your life. You must create time to take care of the whole you: mind, body, and spirit. Try to spend less of that precious time in the sick role, going from doctor to doctor and treatment to treatment, and more of it exploring practices and exercises that boost your vitality and well-being.

My most successful patients are those who can strike a healthy balance between things like work, home life, and relationships on the one hand, and looking after their own needs on the other. Remember: You really can't successfully take care of others if you don't first take great care of yourself. Everyone's situation is unique and ever changing, so I suggest you remain mindful of the balance in your life and adjust things as you go along. Remember: Life is a journey, preferably a long and fulfilling one.

Step Six: Modify Your Environment

A valuable lesson I've learned in treating chronic pain is the importance of a supportive environment. I've found that creating a nurturing and healing environment for my patients at my center helps them take control of their pain and their lives. Unfortunately, when they leave that environment and return home, things can unravel if their home atmosphere lacks the same support. Home life has the potential to really help things along—or play the role of the spoiler.

Chapter 20 provides helpful hints for creating a home environment that can sustain all the wonderful parts of your makeover. This can be a give-and-take process, and one thing that might need to change is you, including how you communicate. Everyone in the home has a role to play in creating the best environment.

Step Seven: Gain Perspective

As you have probably guessed by now, our modern health care system is often a less-than-ideal tool for controlling chronic pain problems. Indeed, as I pointed out earlier, sometimes it can be part of the problem. Be that as it may, modern medicine remains an inherent part of our lives, and it isn't going away any time soon. As a matter of practicality, I recommend that you periodically take a step back and reevaluate your treatments. Are they in-line with your long-term goals? Do they help get you where you want to be, or are they holding up your forward progress?

I realize that learning how to make medicine work for you and not against you can be difficult, especially if you don't have a background in health care. That is why I present important facts and different perspectives to help educate you on all your options. I think when you finish this book many of your questions will have been answered—but new questions will have been raised. That is precisely what I want to see happen! After all, this might be just the beginning of a process for you. Don't hesitate to communicate your thoughts and questions to your doctors. They need your feedback so they can best serve you. As always, I recommend you consult with them before making any wholesale changes in how you manage your health.

Let's face it: For all the problems with our modern health care system, and for the many times it fails to adequately help those with chronic pain, it is still the system we must deal with, so you need to make the best of it.

Let's Get Started!

I suspect you have, without even thinking about it, taken a few hundred breaths while reading this chapter. Now it is time to learn how to use the breath, the first step in your chronic pain makeover.

CHAPTER 11

Breathing

One of the best tools each and every one of us has for managing pain is the *breath*. The simple yet powerful act of breathing, which we typically perform more than seventeen hundred times a day without even thinking about it, can be a potent weapon for working past the pain and regaining control of your life. I realize that what I'm telling you here may make you feel like you just bought a popular cookbook, eagerly opened it, and found that the best cooking tip is to use something as ubiquitous as tap water. But take it from someone who has treated thousands of patients and monitored the long-term effects of just about every treatment imaginable: There are no magic potions or super-duper gadgets that will serve you more admirably than your breath.

Take Control One Breath at a Time

The subject of breathing may, at first glance, seem simple, but I urge you to resist the temptation to gloss over it. Progressing from a "breathing apprentice" to a "breathing expert" requires practice and skill. Though it may seem tedious and trivial, I can assure you that mastering and implementing breathing techniques will bring you one of the greatest rewards imaginable: the gift of *control*. Taking charge of this simple action makes you the captain of your ship once again.

Many of us find ourselves stuck in traffic at one point or another, and some of us slog through thick commuter gravy five days a week getting to work and back. This type of driving can trigger tension and stress, which can manifest as a sore neck, tight shoulders, and a rapid heart rate. We also become "emotionally tense" and agitated, sometimes spitting out choice expletives at the car that just cut us off. We typically assume that our physical and emotional responses are inevitable and unavoidable, but the next time you are caught in terrible traffic, try turning off the radio chatter and focusing on your breath. Pay attention to the slow rise and fall of your belly as you breathe in and out, tuning out all thoughts about what's happening on the road. You may be surprised, but you will certainly be delighted, to discover that not only will your muscles begin to relax and your heart stop pounding, but you will also gain *control of you,* instead of allowing the situation to dictate how your body and mind feel and react.

Remember that you have control over how you breathe, and how you breathe affects you physically and emotionally. This means you always have a pain-managing "medicine" at your disposal, and no one or nothing, including your pain, can take that away from you unless you let it.

The Rhythm of a Beating Diaphragm

Let's review some fundamentals about breathing. For starters, the second-by-second action of inhaling and exhaling air is managed by a very vigilant portion of the brain known as the brain stem, which deals with involuntary activities. Acting on information received from other parts of the nervous system and brain, the brain stem sets a pace or rhythm for the respiratory system to follow.

The brain uses a specific nerve, the *phrenic nerve,* like a telephone line to instruct the diaphragm to contract. Every time it receives "the call," the diaphragm lowers itself, pushing the abdominal muscles out and allowing the lungs to expand and fill with air. Then the diaphragm relaxes, moving back up to its starting position. This allows the abdominal muscles to move back into place, forcing the lungs to push air out. There are also accessory muscles around the ribs and abdomen that help the lungs expand even more and squeeze out extra air upon exhalation. With each inhalation, the lungs bring in oxygen, which moves into the blood so the heart can pump it to all the tissues that need it for energy. With each exhalation the lungs eliminate carbon dioxide, a waste product found in the blood that is produced when our bodies burn fuel.

Think of the diaphragm as a large, flexible dome sitting at the bottom of the rib cage. A large muscle, it helps separate the heart and lungs above, in the thorax (chest cavity), from the intestines, liver, and other organs below, in the abdominal cavity. When the diaphragm contracts, it forces itself down onto the abdomen. This action opens up more space around the lungs. The resulting expansion of the chest creates negative pressure on the lungs, which allows air to flow in from the outside. The diaphragm then moves back up toward the chest as it relaxes. This exerts positive pressure on the lungs, and air is pushed back out.

This back-and-forth motion of air is *rhythmic,* meaning it repeats itself at regular intervals, like the rhythmic beat of music. With music, sound is carried through matter in the form of waves. The waves transfer energy through particles of air to our ears, brains, and, if we get up and dance, to our fingers and toes. The energy released from a musical instrument can move into us and re-create the same pulsating beat inside our bones, connecting us with the instrument. Likewise, the rhythm of breathing involves the transfer of energy back and forth from within us to our external environment.

Have you ever walked down the street and heard a talented street musician playing an instrument? If you are like me, you feel a sense of joy as the harmony resonates within. We humans enjoy calming harmonic motions, whether in the form of waves lapping on the beach or beautiful music. A calming breathing rhythm has the power to improve our outlook in a manner similar to music. When you learn how to use your breath as a form of calming harmonic motion, you can dispel physical tension and emotional stress in the form of energy released through respiration.

We know that stress, acting through the fight-or-flight response, changes our breathing pattern; it becomes quicker and shallower. If we breathe too fast, or hyperventilate, we get dizzy because we are releasing too much carbon dioxide. Rapid breathing can also generate a sense of gasping for air, which creates even more anxiety, makes us breathe ever faster and shallower, triggers more anxiety, and on and on. We also know that the brain stem is part of the pain matrix inside the brain, so deliberately sending the brain positive feedback about breathing will influence what is being "said" inside this matrix. You can do this via the parasympathetic nervous system (PNS). When the PNS becomes more active, you are better able to relax (See chapter 6). Consciously slowing down a respiratory rate accelerated by stress "turns on" the PNS and you start to calm down.

As you can see, breathing can connect the body with the mind, instantaneously linking the involuntary, unconscious mind with active, conscious thoughts. Since our thoughts play an integral role in the emotions we experience, you can use your breath to cut negative thoughts off at the pass before they get a chance to hijack your emotions. Before you know it, your breath can help you short-circuit the chronic pain cycle. (Your breath can also help you kick the road rage habit, getting you to your destination in a much better mental and physical state.)

Time for You to Be With You

At my center, patients spend time in a special room called the Wellness Room, where my staff trains them in meditation, relaxation, and breathing exercises. You might be thinking that I'm a very nice doctor for encouraging my patients to set aside time each day just to chill. It turns out this is often the hardest class for my patients to participate in. Clearing the mind of all other thoughts and focusing on breathing is surprisingly difficult. The brain likes to wander, even toward negative or dysfunctional thoughts. It can be extremely hard to sit still and be calm if your thoughts continue to drift. You run the risk of being afraid to be alone with yourself, which robs you of the opportunity to take advantage of the healing that breathing and meditation or prayer has to offer.

Because we are so accustomed to stimulation from cell phones, computers, televisions, radios, and other sources, we seldom find ourselves alone for quiet time. I think the central nervous system becomes so used to the noise it becomes like an addiction. It starts to crave the noisy stimulation; it needs it to feel "normal." Our minds seem to constantly seek information from e-mails, text messages, and television shows. This makes it all the more important to be disciplined about shutting off these tempting distractions and giving your brain the time it needs to help heal both mind and body. I tell my patients that there are many ways to do this, including switching off the cell phone and taking a short walk, turning off the TV and reading a good book, or playing board games with their children or grandchildren. Technology is not going to vanish and it is not inherently bad for us, but you need to contain it in order to optimize your physical and emotional well-being.

In chapter 5, I shared a valuable concept with you when I discussed the great importance of contact time, which is the amount of time patients spend in comprehensive treatment programs. The evidence tells us that intensive programs with lots of contact time provide numerous valuable, long-lasting results. If you recall, I connected that contact-time dot to you, the reader, imploring you to carefully decide how you spend your time each day.

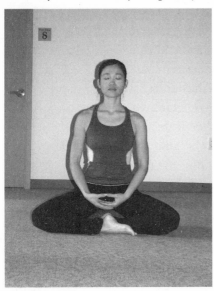

Mastering the art of therapeutic breathing requires lots of contact time, which means you have to devote time to mastering it. My patients don't just walk in the Wellness Room, dash through two minutes of breathing exercises, and then walk out. They spend about an hour per session with one of our wellness instructors doing some of the exercises you will read about here. Take a moment to consider which breathing and meditation practice would best fit into your day and commit yourself to it. It doesn't matter whether you practice in the morning, in the afternoon, in the evening, or at night, as long as you create a space in your day, every day, to let breathing nourish you to a greater vitality.

Getting Started

One well-founded, time-honored approach to breathing, called diaphragmatic breathing, involves relaxing the belly during inhalation. The first step in diaphragmatic breathing involves thinking about the belly during breathing. Lie flat on your back and observe how it rises during inhalation and falls naturally during exhalation. Notice how much easier it is to breathe when the belly is relaxed. Try tensing it and see how much harder it feels to move air in and out of the lungs. The softer the abdomen gets, the more the lungs can fill with air and breathing shifts from shallow to deep. This change is easier to appreciate if you put your hand on your belly and feel it move back and forth.

Try these easy steps to become acquainted with diaphragmatic breathing:

1. Sit down or lie flat on your back in a quiet place.
2. Close your eyes.
3. Concentrate on the motion of the belly.
4. If your mind wanders—and it will—reconnect with the motion of the belly and movement of the breath.
5. See if you can do this for at least five minutes.

Now take this concept into your daily life. When you feel yourself becoming tense or angry, wait a moment. Place your hand on your belly and become aware of the motion. Concentrate on this motion for several breaths, and then ask yourself how you feel. The negative emotions you just had should be mostly gone as you become more relaxed.

You can use breathing exercises to do more than quiet the mind: They can also stimulate the mind and boost mental clarity. You don't have to rely on a double, extra-hot vanilla latte to get you there! Try the following exercise when you wake up in the morning:

1. Sit up tall with your eyes closed and your tongue up against the roof of your mouth.
2. Breathe in and out very quickly through your nose with your mouth closed.
3. Notice the pumping sensation taking place at your abdomen while you do this breathing. This means some of those accessory muscles are active.
4. You will hear noise as the air is rapidly pushed in and out.
5. At first you may not be able to breathe this way for more than about fifteen seconds, but it will get easier with practice. Practice this exercise for a few minutes each morning.

I personally find this exercise helpful when I wake up anxious about the day ahead and need to calm myself down so that I can focus on what is important and reduce excess nervous tension. Not only do I work full-time in a busy medical practice, but I am also a self-employed small-business owner responsible for things like rent and payroll. This special breathing exercise is one tool that helps prevent the typical daily stressors we all face from overloading my coping circuits so that I can still focus my attention on my patients, or even family, when they need me.

Because the diaphragm is a large muscle, it helps to warm it up before exercising it, just as you do other muscles. I remember participating in a workshop that strongly advocated doing just that. They put a group of us in a room and had us all belt out "huh, huh, huh . . ." Try it; you'll warm up your diaphragm *and* give your neighbors' eardrums a good workout at 6:00 a.m.

Exercising Your Breath

Let me share with you some of the other breathing exercises my patients learn in the Wellness Room. Most of these come from Eastern practices, including yoga, which you will learn more about in chapter 17. We often use relaxing rhythmic music during these sessions. Feel free to pick music that works for you; we all have different tastes.

Sun and Moon Breathing

This exercise involves alternating breaths between the nostrils. Use one hand to gently close the right nostril. Exhale through the left nostril, then inhale. Now, with the same hand, release your right nostril and gently seal your left nostril. Exhale and then inhale through the right. Now back to the other side. You can continue this exercise for five minutes or longer. In yogic tradition, the left side represents the energy of the moon, while the right side is the energy of the sun. Consider using this for help with stress, anxiety, unwanted cravings, and even headaches.

The Body Scan

This breathing technique also engages the mind in some thoughtful meditation. When you feel overwhelmed by pain, use it as a tool to try to put your pain in a "box." In other words, do not allow your pain to identify with the real you. Here's how to do it:

1. Lie on your back with your arms and legs outstretched.
2. Close your eyes and become aware of your belly's movement with each inhalation and exhalation.
3. Draw your attention first to your left foot. Breathe into and out of it for a few moments. Visualize the air moving down to and expanding into the foot as you inhale; then imagine the foot relaxing as the air flows out of it during exhalation.
4. Slowly make your way all the way up your body, "breathing into" each part of your body in succession.
5. As you leave each body part or section, let it go from your mind and redirect your attention to the next part.
6. When your attention is drawn to a painful part of the body, avoid becoming judgmental. Instead of creating opinions about the pain, simply recognize its presence while you breathe.

Thirty-five-year-old Natalie suffered for years with a great deal of neck pain, even after trying many treatments, medicines, and an extensive four-level cervical fusion in her neck. Unfortunately, even after all of this, her pain continued and her neck got as stiff as a board. In fact, her neck became so immobile that she was unable to shampoo her own hair or otherwise groom herself, and driving was out of the question. Having suffered through many failed treatments, she was amazed to see how much the body scan helped her situation. It took her a few weeks to get comfortable making it a part of her regular routine, but now it has become a great tool to relax tight muscles in her neck and shoulders so she can move her neck more freely and with less pain. The body scan has also made it easier for her to drift off to sleep at bedtime as well as get back to sleep, instead of tossing and turning, in the middle of the night.

Exhaling First
Exhaling before you begin a breathing exercise forces you to engage accessory muscles around your ribs and abdomen as you blow the air out. (Think about squeezing the air out of an inflatable beach ball; imagine these muscles are your fingers pressing in on the beach ball.) Reversing your breathing pattern by exhaling first also makes you much more aware of your breath. This should increase the amount of air you move in and out of the lungs and restore calmness. Try this exercise for a few minutes every day.

Awakening the PSN
I have extolled the virtues of inducing the parasympathetic nervous system (PNS) as a way to reduce stress and anxiety and manage pain. This breathing exercise will help boost parasympathetic tone (discussed in chapter 6):

1. Inhale through your nose with your mouth closed and your tongue raised to the roof of your mouth.
2. After a full inhalation, hold your breath for five counts, or whatever length of time feels right.

3. Exhale deeply out the mouth. This typically creates a noise as the air is pushed out . . . *hhhhhaaaaahhhhh.*

Try doing this for three to five minutes at a time. Don't feel you have to go the full five minutes. Do it as long as you comfortably can. Some people have trouble getting started with this exercise and even feel a little light-headed in the beginning. So start slowly, and make sure you're sitting down when you begin.

Monitoring Your Body and Mind

My wellness instructors have also found this exercise to be a useful tool for clearing the mind of negative emotions and thoughts. I find it especially helpful in times of stress.

1. Get into a comfortable, erect sitting posture with your eyes closed. Silently ask yourself what thoughts and feelings you are experiencing. Acknowledge those feelings; pain might be one of them.
2. Become aware of your breath, including the flow of air into and out of your body. Try to adopt a state of stillness.
3. Now expand your awareness to include your whole body—your shoulders, pelvis, back, jaw, and so on. What is present in your whole body at that moment? Pain? Tightness? Tingling?
4. What hidden emotions do you recognize?
5. It may take you five to ten minutes to work your way through all of the steps.

"Breathing Down" the Pain

When we are in pain we have a tendency to breathe hard, but doing so only makes the pain more intense and the breathing motion harder to perform. As you begin to engage your body more, draw your mind into this process by linking the two together with the power of your breath. If your pain starts to get worse or flares up, let your thoughts gravitate toward your breath and practice some of the simple exercises above. Learn from what has just happened. Did you try to do too much too quickly? Could you have avoided the flare-up by pacing yourself better? Were parts of you overly tense? Next time you perform the activity that triggered the pain, try using your breath as a way to relax yourself and see if it becomes easier.

Hang in There

Being mindful of the breath is not just an exercise to practice at isolated times in your own personal Wellness Room. You want to bring mindful breathing into your daily life, making it a part of what you do when you're talking to an angry customer, waiting in line at baggage check, cooking dinner, or exercising at the gym. (Appropriate breathing during exercise can make a big difference. Exhale during the motion and inhale as you rest. Try doing the same exercise while holding your breath and you will see how much harder it is.)

Practicing the breathing exercises I described here and making them a routine part of daily life provides immediate benefits for many people. They learn how to use the breath to handle their emotions, manage pain flare-ups, and perform exercises more comfortably. Unfortunately, some people may have to work harder than others to master breathing. This doesn't mean they're doing anything "bad" or "wrong," for keeping the mind focused on the breath doesn't come naturally to most of us. It may take time before some can feel that mindful breathing is reducing flare-ups of pain or negative emotions. Remember: My patients spend many hours mastering breathing and wellness exercises, and they also spend time with my staff getting more hands-on education as they learn how to use the breath while doing functional activities like exercising. I can tell you that while most struggle with this process, over time the majority find it immensely helpful, and you will too, if you are able to stick with it.

I understand that it can be difficult and feel awkward to learn how to use your breath; it certainly takes a little getting used to. But if you practice it every day for a few weeks, it will become second nature. And once you develop mindful breathing and meditation habits, you'll find yourself releasing negative thoughts and feelings. This is important as we move into the subject of acceptance.

CHAPTER 12

Acceptance: Your Path to Happiness

When Melanie was just a girl, doctors discovered that she had scoliosis, a congenital curvature of the spine that can cause pain, fatigue, nerve damage, arthritis, and other problems. Her parents had arranged for her to undergo corrective surgery when she was young, and she managed to function relatively well into adulthood, although she still had some pain. Unfortunately, Melanie could not accept the fact that her spine did not look and feel "normal." And as far as she was concerned, dealing with pain every day was not an option. So when Melanie became an adult, she underwent a series of surgeries with the hope of "fixing" her spine. Unfortunately, each one seemed to trigger new problems. The long hours of being in a fixed position during these surgeries caused new injuries to other parts of her body. All the cutting and probing caused scar tissue to develop around her nerves and spine, producing inflammation and pain, and she literally shrunk in size. As far as I can tell, all of this treatment only made matters worse, and her pain medications seemed to stop working to boot (another case of opioid-induced hyperalgesia).

Melanie is a beautiful woman and a dedicated mother with a lot to offer. She's always kind and cheerful with others, never mean or angry. Unfortunately, I don't think she has ever adequately appreciated her many gifts because she dwells so much on her imperfections. Her difficulty accepting a health problem that was inherited and not preventable created more suffering than she ever bargained for.

This book is all about taking charge and regaining control, so it may seem odd that I'm devoting an entire chapter to the subject of acceptance. *Acceptance* is practically a dirty word: When many of my patients hear the word, they cringe because they think it means giving up, losing the battle against chronic pain. They wonder how they can possibly be in control of their pain and their lives if they accept the very thing that is causing them so much pain, literally and figuratively. It *is* a counterintuitive concept, yet I have seen how resisting pain can cause even more emotional suffering and torment and add new layers of suffering. The reality is that those who refuse to accept their pain can find that it continues to grow. The people I see in my office who have *not* accepted the situation are like volcanoes about to explode; their emotions are constantly smoldering below the surface, about to blow. When the emotions start to fly, they are usually of the types that seem to make the pain worse—rage, agitation, and guilt.

The Five Stages of Grief

Elizabeth Kubler-Ross, MD, was a Swiss doctor who devoted her career to caring for the terminally ill. In her groundbreaking book, *On Death and Dying,* she explained her theories about the cycle of grieving. When people learn that they are dying, they go through five basic stages of grief:

1. *Denial:* "This can't be happening to me."
2. *Anger:* "I really got shafted this time!"
3. *Bargaining:* "I'll do anything to get rid of this problem."
4. *Depression:* "I don't want to go out of my room."
5. *Acceptance:* "I can deal with this."

These five stages of grief can be applied to other catastrophic losses as well, including divorce, unemployment, and the loss of a loved one, as well as the experience of chronic pain. Yes, to develop chronic pain is to suffer loss: You may lose the ability to sleep through the night, work, play, and maintain relationships. You lose your faith in your body and perhaps in yourself. You lose your sense of well-being, physically as well as emotionally. You lose your feeling that you are in control of your life and will never be a burden on your family. You lose the feeling that all is right with the world. These are terrible losses that must be dealt with.

Kubler-Ross felt that people had to process, or work through, each stage as it arose or else they could become stuck and unable to move forward toward acceptance. Unfortunately, there are no societal or religious processes to help us grieve the losses that come with chronic pain. That's why I have seen so many chronic pain patients mired in their grief, unable to accept and let go.

Obstacles to Grieving Chronic Pain

My behavioral health staff can usually help figure out which of the five stages seem to be retarding someone's progress. By the time patients make it through my door, they're usually stuck in either anger or depression.

One such patient was Jack, a forty-two-year-old accountant who seemed to be angry about absolutely everything. He kept getting treatment after treatment, but he never felt it was enough and certainly not as much as he deserved. He had issues with everybody and everything. At every appointment he complained to me about something else he hadn't received but *knew* he deserved. He'd always start the same way: "I can't believe I didn't get . . ." Finally, after several years had gone by, he came in one day and said, "I can't believe my wife kicked me out!"

Well, the man's poor wife had finally had enough of his complaining, which stemmed from his anger. Jack remained angry for years because he was focused on getting more and more treatment and would not accept the situation for what it was. He never tried to figure out how to make the best of things, which means that nothing could ever satisfy him and relieve his anger.

Unable to work through the stages of grief, many people never reach the acceptance they need to manage their pain and improve the quality of their lives. This refusal to accept the reality of chronic pain can take many forms. For example, people may have difficulty with the following:

- *Accepting that an injury has taken place.* Perhaps a nerve in the hand was damaged in an accident, making fine motor activities a struggle. Refusal to acknowledge that damage has occurred can lead to refusal to rehabilitate the muscles and nerves.

- *Acknowledging the need for change in daily activities.* This might mean insisting on doing all the things they always did, such as lifting heavy objects or playing strenuous weekend basketball, despite great pain.
- *Understanding that their lives may have to undergo major change.* This could take the form of not accepting that their pain will prevent them from continuing to work in their current position, avoiding retraining, and neglecting to look for a new job. It might also mean refusing to accept treatment or help with their activities from friends and family.
- *Accepting that the pain is a chronic problem.* They may be wholly committed to finding a "cure" that will make all their pain go away. Lots of problems can be created through the belief that someone or something, somewhere, will eventually solve everything if one just keeps looking. This desperate search and willingness to undergo any and all "cures" can lead to terrible problems. Remember: One of the biggest contributors to the pain I treat each day is the aftereffects of past medical treatments that wound up making things worse, not better. Countless people put themselves through a wringer because they're not ready to accept that their pain can't be fixed. They also can't accept that they must take responsibility for and manage their own pain. They say things like, "It's not my fault I was hit by the other car. I shouldn't have to be the one to deal with all of this pain. Surely *somebody* out there can *fix* me!"

Too often I see people who were injured at work go on disability and eventually lose their jobs because they simply cannot go back to them, or the job has been given to someone else. But they don't move on mentally; they don't say, "OK, I don't have this job anymore, so I need to find a new job or get into a whole new line of work." They're stuck and they remain stuck; they can't make the transition. They understand the situation intellectually; they tell me, "I don't have the job anymore." But they don't accept it.

Patients who never arrive at the stage of acceptance often wind up full of stitches, screws, and plates, which cause more scar tissue to form, sometimes in places where other tissues are most vulnerable. Lives may be put on hold for weeks, months, or even years while patients try to recover or wait for some expected outcome. The many medicines they take can cause constipation, sedation, poor memory, and in some cases increased levels of pain. These side effects prompt many to reach out for more of the same kind of help, and the patients dig themselves into deeper and deeper holes. Meanwhile they often harm themselves financially and, whether or not the money lasts, their families inevitably suffer.

Although many people fear that acceptance means giving up, in truth it can be the absence of acceptance that holds everything up. Nonacceptance causes lots of busy energy but no forward progress, and it can make people stick grimly to certain courses of action that they cannot see are useless.

Letting Go of Resistance

Accepting the fact that you currently experience pain is *not* the same thing as accepting the fact that you will continue to suffer. Accepting is not the problem; resisting is. It is the act of resistance that brings about the most negative feelings, that creates turbulence to the flow of nature. This type of upstream swimming is taxing and carries you away from where you want to go. It keeps you reaching out for treatments that will always be ineffective.

A yoga posture called Pigeon Pose helps illustrate how the body responds when it's resisting pain. To get into this pose, you do something like the splits with your front leg bent at the knee and placed under you; then you lie forward over the bent leg while the other leg points straight back behind you. The pressure from stretching the muscles and tendons on the outside of the hip and thigh can be intense, and the more the body resists the stretch, the tighter the muscles get. But when you breathe and "let go" of these same muscles, the body folds deeper into the stretch, releasing the tension stored in these muscles.

When the body is challenged or stressed—and pain is a powerful stressor—it naturally wants to tighten and resist the movement. That's exactly when the mind must consciously recognize what's happening and ask the body to relax, which will allow a much better stretch.

Letting Go by Being Thankful

I have found that one of the best ways to arrive at acceptance is to turn your focus away from your pain and toward all the good things in your life. I tell my patients to

- Take some time to think about what you have to be thankful for: your wonderful kids, your loving spouse/partner, your friends, the great experiences you have had, your hobbies, your religion, and everything else in your life that's good. Take some time every day to think about what you have to be thankful for.
- Appreciate yourself and what you've accomplished when working through your chronic pain challenges. Pat yourself on the back and congratulate yourself for the great progress you've made.
- Be happy with yourself. Love yourself.

It's very helpful to keep track of the good things in your life in a journal. Write something in it every day, jot down something you have to be thankful for, keep track of the things you've done that day that you can congratulate yourself for. Maybe you were able to cook a special dinner for the first time in six months, or you made someone else laugh. Keep track of your progress, and congratulate yourself for each and every positive step along the way.

Here are a few examples of affirmations that help with acceptance from some of the folks I have worked with:

- From a computer programmer: "I know I can't do as much keyboarding as I used to, but with my knowledge and experience, and with the right adjustments, I have a lot to offer my company."

- From a competitive triathlete: "Even though my body can't take the pounding anymore, I am thankful for entering a few competitions a year—not to win, but to see good friends that I made along the way."

- From a breadwinning parent: "I used to always feel guilty about not being able to play ball with my kids, but now I know the important thing is that I spend time with them."

- From a vice president of marketing: "I know that I can manage the pain that I have, even if it doesn't go away."

- From a full-time mom: "It's hard but I do my best to balance my time carefully so that there is still time left over for me to take care of me."

- From a lady who is looking for work: "I'm really proud of myself. I paced myself, but I still finished the charity walk for breast cancer."

Accepting and Taking Flight

Just as the acknowledgment and letting go of resistance is a key step to achieving a better stretch, it's also a key step in achieving pain relief. And because the act of resistance is usually unconscious, you have to consciously think about letting go or you may continue to hold yourself back without realizing it.

When patients with debilitating chronic pain problems finally reach acceptance, the transformation they experience is so powerful, it's obvious to everyone. One day they look troubled and tormented, but the next they may exhibit a glow of calm and peace, because they know they are going to be okay. The pain hasn't magically disappeared, but the torment has. Worry has been replaced by confidence in themselves and in their ability to manage their pain.

If you don't feel this sense of confidence and inner tranquility, you may be refusing to accept your pain. Timing is often key: I have seen folks stuck in resistance for months or even years. But once they were ready, the transformation they experienced was nothing short of miraculous. Similarly, what you get out of this book will depend on your level of readiness. And what you glean from it today may be different from what you glean if you come back to it in the future, because we are all ever-evolving creatures.

An elderly woman named Mary learned to accept her pain after undergoing seven spine surgeries. She injured her back while in the military and is now retired. By the time I saw her, she had reached the stage of acceptance. She comes to my office periodically for "fine-tuning," always relaxed and happy. Although she still has a lot of physical issues, she never pressures me to "fix" her. Instead, she gives me advice on how to raise my children! To tell you the truth, I look forward to her visits, because she makes me feel better about life.

So continue to nourish your body, mind, and spirit with healthy things, and when your time comes to fly, you will soar. In the next chapter, we'll learn how engaging the creative side of the brain can help release feelings bottled up inside that may be preventing you from reaching important stages like acceptance.

CHAPTER 13
Art Imitating Pain

The brain is an adaptable organ, ready and willing to change and grow when called upon. Its millions of tiny cells are constantly on alert for messages from the nervous system, ready to react to them. Imagine being at a cocktail party full of tipsy, chattering, social butterflies. As soon as one person at the party tells another about a scandalous rumor, the story spreads like wildfire through the room until practically everyone is talking about it. Our neurons are like those partygoers, always on the lookout for a good story, and once they get hold of it, they make sure the brain knows about it.

We learned earlier that nerve cells in the brain can grow and develop in the presence of the right type of stimulation, even at advanced ages. The hippocampus, an area of the brain that plays an important part in learning and memory, can expand its neuron resources (create new neurons, or nerve cells) to help you learn new things, but only if you challenge it to do so. We call this process of sprouting new neurons *neurogenesis*. Exposing the mind to new and provocative activities helps stimulate neurogenesis. On the other hand, stress hormones like cortisol, impair the process.

Earlier I suggested that you can use the mind as a tool to promote healing and recovery. This chapter looks at an intriguing way to tap into the creative resources of the brain to help heal the wounds of chronic pain.

As a newly minted pain doctor, I attended a presentation on art therapy at a prestigious cancer center. (Coincidently, it was the same center where I had been taught years before to wake people from surgery with no pain.) Specially trained therapists showed us how they used art to help grieving children who had lost family members to cancer. I was stunned by the feelings these youngsters expressed through the pictures they created. Using colors and shapes applied to paper, they revealed emotions that would never have come out

151

through mere words. I remembered that during my own adolescent and teenage years, when trapped in moments of awkwardness and shyness, I enjoyed the creative freedom of drawing and painting.

If art therapy is a useful way to help children and adults overcome catastrophic events like death, addiction, and abuse, it seemed to me that it should be able to help folks struggling to overcome the devastations of chronic pain. Surprisingly, practically nothing had been published on the use of art therapy for chronic pain. Still, when my partner and I started our first comprehensive pain program, we jumped at the chance of bringing on an art therapist. We knew we couldn't restore painful bodies without healing afflicted minds and spirits, and we wanted to give our patients every opportunity to succeed.

Please keep in mind that many of my patients are blue-collar workers who were first injured lifting a ton of bricks or driving a truck. Most have not been asked to do anything "creative" since they were in grade school. Our typical patient does not walk into his or her first art therapy session saying, "Wow, I can't wait to get started!" Believe me, many of our patients begin with the same skepticism that you are probably experiencing right now. You won't be the first person to say, "But I'm not an artist, so this can't help me."

Creative Healers

I remember how much John struggled with art therapy during his first two weeks. He was a very large auto mechanic, weighing close to three hundred pounds, who hurt his back at work and had been on disability for a few years. During one of his first art therapy classes, this large man turned red, jumped out of his seat, stormed into the bathroom, and refused to come out. We later learned that he was never in touch with his feelings, even way back in childhood. He had always dealt with stress by drinking beer and had resolved conflicts with others by punching them in the nose. This was the first time in his life he had tried to connect with his emotions, and it was so scary the first time around that he ran to the bathroom for cover!

Not only did my terrified patient eventually come around to full participation in art therapy, he changed his whole persona. Over time John became noticeably calmer and more cheerful, and he regained enough strength to resume working again. It's impossible, of course, to determine exactly how much the art therapy contributed to his recovery, but I'm certain that it played a significant role in helping him process emotions like depression and anxiety. In the end John was very proud of the changes he saw in himself, changes that only occurred because he opened his mind and challenged it.

The reason that patients like John benefit from art therapy, whether or not they are "good artists," is *it is the process of creation that matters,* not what the final product looks like. The creative mind needs to focus and filter out the background noise. The creative process of art therapy engages the parasympathetic nervous system, which helps reduce pain and stress, and also helps process conflicts hidden in the unconscious mind. Emotions can also be hidden away in various parts of the body, causing additional pain. We can't always discover them just by talking. Sometimes we have to discover them through processes like art therapy that encourage emotional exploration.

People communicate in different ways. Some are very verbal and can easily express their feelings. Others, who prefer to read or listen, may not communicate as well. For many, engaging in a creative process like art therapy can be a means of tapping into feelings that otherwise would be missed. Patients often comment on how difficult it is to describe their chronic pain experience in words. I frequently find that they feel isolated and alone because they haven't been able to express their true feelings to their friends and family. The greater the variety of tools for expression at their disposal, the easier it is for them to work through areas of distress.

In 1925 a young woman named Frida Kahlo was seriously injured in a bus accident that left her with chronic pain for the rest of her life. While in the hospital she learned to paint and used art as a way to express her feelings about pain. Kahlo eventually became a famous early twentieth-century artist. Some of her best-known works are self-portraits that depict symbolic expressions of her pain.

Left to Right, Closed to Open

The brain is divided into two halves: the right and left hemispheres. The different sections of the brain (e.g., the cortex and brain stem) occupy both hemispheres. The two hemispheres are connected and communicate through a structure known as the *corpus collosum*. There are some basic distinctions between the two hemispheres worth noting. You are probably already aware that someone who is right handed is considered left-brain dominant. That's because activities involving one side of the body are predominantly engineered on the opposite side of the brain. So if you rely more on your right hand, you also rely more on your left brain for all kinds of activities, including writing, opening doors, and brushing your teeth.

Regardless of which hand you prefer to use, the two hemispheres seem to specialize in certain areas. Language, for example, is more of a left-brain function. That's why strokes and other injuries to the left side of the brain are more likely to affect speech than are injuries to the right side. The left side also focuses on more analytical functions like calculations and logic. The right hemisphere, however, is more involved in artistic pursuits. The right side pays more attention to things like the prosody (rhythm and tone) of speech or music, intuition, comparisons, and visual processing.

A man named David came to my center with a fifteen-year history of chronic low back pain. During that time, he underwent a total of three spinal surgeries, the last a fusion involving hardware implants. He was a classic example of a patient being told that if he didn't have the surgery, he could end up in a wheelchair. Unfortunately, David's pain never went away, and he slid into a deep depression. Trying to work became so physically and emotionally exhausting that he had to stop and get help.

David was an engineer, and a very analytical one at that. His mind was always occupied with formulas and calculations. In other words, he was about as left-brained as they come. He was used to pushing his emotions away and "just working through things," but his pain and depression became too overpowering to handle this way.

When David came to his first art therapy session, he immediately announced, "I can't draw!" His first project was to find pictures in magazines that expressed aspects of what he was going through. Begrudgingly at first, David found some pictures that symbolized emotional aspects of his pain, including anger and depression. These were his dominant emotions, and he had never been able to talk about them in the past. David noted, "As time went on, I became more expressive. I started to connect the different images together in ways that mirrored the way my life was connected—my wife, career, back pain, and so on—during bad moments."

As the weeks progressed, David began to feel "opened." Talking about his art projects to the other patients was very therapeutic, whereas talking directly about topics like pain and anger had been too awkward and difficult before. "Everything in your program was great," he said later, "but art was my defining moment. It helped me get rid of my demons. I was always very analytical but never creative, even though I appreciated looking at nice works of art. Letting go of my analytical side helped me tap into my hidden creative mind."

Over the years countless patients have told me about cognitive problems, like lapses in memory, that had become a part of their chronic pain experience. Many have described a feeling of mental cloudiness that contrasted with the sharp thoughts they were accustomed to. I asked David if he had had a similar experience, and it turns out he had. He described a sensation of "wearing cloudy glasses that were out of focus" since his pain had begun. I imagined this was distressing for a brainy engineer. Indeed he had been frequently embarrassed about missing social engagements or forgetting things his friends had told him. I was curious to know how engaging the untapped creative side of his brain would affect his mental clarity. Several months after David started art therapy, he found his memory had definitely improved. His mind still wasn't as sharp as it once had been, and he still forgot things like appointments on occasion, but he was very pleased with the improvement.

David was kind enough to share some of his personal creations to help illustrate what types of projects you can do at home.

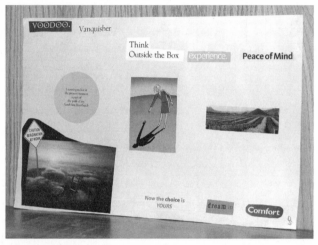

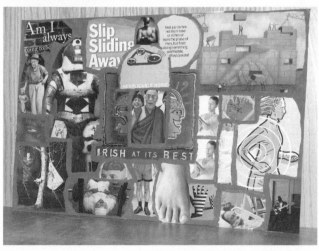

The Mozart Effect

Drawing isn't the only art form that is believed to improve cognition. Music therapy, for example, is successfully used for stroke recovery. In 1991, French researcher Alfred A. Tomatis, MD, claimed that listening to Mozart actually promoted brain development, and he dubbed the phenomenon the Mozart Effect. This led to the controversial notion that Mozart's music could actually boost intelligence and IQ, an idea that many scientists now believe is overstated. But that didn't stop Zell Miller, governor of Georgia, from requesting an annual budget of $105,000 in 1998 to purchase a classical music CD for every baby born in the state. Ode to Joy!

Your Homework

Christine Hirabayashi, who has been the art therapist at my center for the last five years, has done literally thousands of art projects with chronic pain sufferers. She notes, "It is hard to filter emotions through art." It can uncork bottled-up feelings by sneaking past our usual defenses. For example, the creative process of gathering pictures that identify with emotions like depression can bring out aspects of the depression that would not be considered or expressed otherwise. It's a way of getting around roadblocks that our brains naturally put up to protect us from certain feelings that are difficult to process.

As Hirabayashi sees it, art creates a direct link between emotions and the unconscious mind. If we have difficulty acknowledging certain feelings and letting them out, then the art projects designed to facilitate this release must take place in a very safe and comforting environment. She recommends this process take place under the supervision of an art therapist who can maintain a supportive atmosphere. She also finds that working in a group offers special support, allowing those working through similar issues to share their experiences, as opposed to communicating only with friends or family members who don't have pain. Hirabayashi says,

"Patients often connect to the images in other peoples' artwork. This helps them realize that they are not the only ones experiencing sadness, fear, and anxiety."

Although a group setting is best, if you do not have access to one, you can work on your own. Here are some things you can do independently, at home, to tap in to your creative healing mind:

- Build an environment in which you will feel safe thinking and working. Your art therapy area should be a place where there is no judgment, no critique of your art. If you have a quiet room, a home office, or other personal space, make it your own and ask family members to stay out. If you must use a common area like a corner of the kitchen, ask family members to respect your privacy and avoid passing judgments on what you create.
- Gather your supplies. There are many different mediums you can use, including all types of paints, crayons, colored pencils, and markers. Find magazines that have pictures that you can clip that illustrate your emotional states. Make sure you have plenty of paper, glue, and other art supplies.
- Consider working with watercolors. Watercolors are harder to control than other types of media; the colors have a tendency to move and bleed on the paper. Allowing yourself to let the paint flow like this can help you let go of pent-up emotions.
- Set the tone. When you work, create a peaceful environment by playing relaxing music.
- Assemble a symbol for balance in your life. Use the mediums of your choice to show what grounds you. This could be an image of a relaxing place like the beach or a forest, pictures of your children, or something more symbolic like a spiritual icon.
- Create a symbol for strength. This can include both physical and emotional strength. Your symbol might include motivational quotes, images of heroic people, and spiritual icons. Look at it often to reinforce your sense of strength.

- Keep an art journal in which you can draw, doodle, or make collages on a regular basis as a form of release.
- Do the Bridge Project: Create a picture that symbolizes where you are now and where you see yourself going.
- Avoid judging what your pictures look like; doing so will help you learn to clear the noise from your mind and live in the moment.

If you'd like to have an art therapist guide you through the process, take a look at the Art Therapy Complete page on my Web site: www.bapwc.com/sub/index.jsp?contentid=zannQ4K1PuETbQmb 3NSSW1sH. You'll also find links to art therapy organizations that may be able to help you.

Always remember it is the process, not the final product, that's important. Your goal is to explore and express your emotions, not create something that pleases an art teacher. If your art opens you up and helps you access and process negative emotions, you have created a masterpiece.

CHAPTER 14
Facing Addiction

"Do the difficult things while they are easy and do the great things while they are small. A journey of a thousand miles must begin with a single step."
—Lao Tzu, ancient Chinese philosopher

It seems like the list of addictive substances grows every year. When I was a boy, smoking was the big bugaboo, because it was both addictive and the cause of deadly diseases like lung cancer. Excessive alcohol intake was considered harmful, as were popular drugs of the era like heroin. There were a few more items on the addiction list, but it was fairly small by today's standards, as people are said to be addicted to all kinds of things, including shopping, eating, gambling, stealing, sex, video games, exercise, caffeine, surfing the Internet, and pornography.

Why is someone who exercises endlessly, drinks loads of coffee, or plays online poker for hours considered an addict, while someone else with exactly the same "hobbies" is just fine? What are the defining characteristics of an addiction?

An addiction is an uncontrolled obsession that is in some way harmful. Smoking (which is actually nicotine addiction) can easily become a dangerous obsession that can damage the respiratory and cardiovascular systems. Compulsive gambling can cause financial ruin. Alcoholism and drug dependency can destroy relationships, careers, and life itself.

Another defining characteristic of addiction is withdrawal, which occurs when access to the addictive substance or activity is interrupted. The symptoms of withdrawal usually include agitation and distress, feelings that can be so unsettling that they force the addict to actively and even aggressively seek what's missing in order to feel normal again. An addiction can fool you into believing that the substance or activity is "a part of who you are," while withdrawal can cause intense mental and physical anguish.

Of course, not all addictions produce consequences as dramatic as terminal illness or financial ruin. I see people every day who have emotional addictions, which may manifest as a constant state of depression, drama seeking, or a clinging to fears and anxieties. Unfortunately, no matter how hard I try to reason with people caught in the grip of an emotional addiction, no matter how many times I explain that their dysfunctional thoughts are causing negative emotions, they have difficulty breaking free. Just as genetics may predispose certain people toward developing chemical dependencies, an emotional predisposition may incline others toward emotional addictions, especially if they aren't vigilant about their thoughts.

Marla, a fifty-three-year-old account executive, came into my office complaining about persistent depression and backaches that never seemed to go away. After we had spoken for a while, it came out that she was furious about an insulting remark one of her coworkers had made to her about her work habits some *five years earlier.* Marla told me she was still just as upset about that incident as she had been the day it occurred. Her brain was so accustomed to thinking about how mad she was that she couldn't shut it off. For Marla, feeling angry had become a part of feeling normal, just as the effect of a shot of heroin feels normal to a heroin addict. And even after Marla understood the adverse impact the anger was having on her mind and body, she couldn't let it go, any more than a smoker could quit cigarettes cold turkey. She was addicted to the negative emotion. For some, letting go of such binding thoughts may require the help of a specially trained therapist or counselor.

Addiction and Chronic Pain: Randal's Story

I've noticed that for many patients the process of recovery doesn't begin until they hit rock bottom. It's as if they need to see what the bottom looks like before they can begin looking up. Most of the patients I see at my center who are suffering from a chemical dependency have no history of alcohol or drug abuse. Typically they sought medical treatment for their pain and wound up becoming dependent on prescribed painkillers.

One of my patients, Randal, had never even flirted with alcohol or drug addiction before a doctor prescribed Norco for his back pain. In fact, he had worked hard to get healthy, dropping 145 excess pounds and getting in great physical shape. He fell in love, married, had two sons, and felt like he was on top of the world. Then he suffered a fall and severely injured his lower back. This gave him a horrible sense of loss, shattered his self-esteem, and left him feeling every single day like he let his family down.

Randal began taking prescribed opioid pain pills, the typical route taken by doctors and patients when they can't seem to get the pain under control. At first this helped dull his pain, but after six months it started to dull Randal. His condition continued to deteriorate, and about five years later he was taking eight pain pills a day. He told me, "The Norco changed me. It took my emotions away, made me feel lethargic about everything, about my whole life." Randal lost faith in himself and in his future, lost the motivation to take care of himself, and started to put on the pounds again.

Randal's descent continued. He lost interest in his family, his job, and himself. He hit rock bottom some two years later when his ever-worsening back condition caused a loss of sexual function and sensation in his legs. At that point Randal felt his life was over. He went into a shell, and he began eating dinner alone in his room and going to sleep immediately afterward. To increase the emotional distance between himself and his family, he became increasingly angry. "I wanted to make everyone hate me so they would feel relieved when I was no longer around," he told me.

Every time Randal tried to go without his pain pills, he only grew meaner. He now recognizes that the only person he was unhappy with was himself. Because he felt so unworthy as a husband and a father, he hid behind the emotional dullness created by his painkillers, and anytime anyone tried to get inside, he chased them away by snarling at them.

Despite the fact that he was taking four to five painkillers upon waking each morning, and an equally large dose at night, Randall's entire body hurt. He had his gallbladder removed because of frequent stomachaches, but that didn't solve the problem. Panic attacks started waking him at 4:00 a.m., the time when the medication levels in his blood fell to low levels. When I met Randal, his wife had just asked him to leave and he was living at his brother's house, sleeping on the couch.

Once I got Randal weaned off of Norco, he changed before my very eyes. He "woke up" emotionally and started to work on the suppressed feelings related to his injury that had been silenced for several years. His motivation returned, and he began to exercise and lose weight. Best of all, he began to like himself again. Randal is now working full-time once more and furthering his career. The original problem, his back pain, is still there, but it's milder and much easier to handle. Randal manages his pain with exercise, breathing, walking, and communicating his feelings effectively. In other words, he manages the pain—not the other way around.

Unfortunately, Randal is still pained by the dissolution of his marriage and the fact that he no longer gets to see his sons every day. He has become much healthier physically, but the scars of his past still linger. He knew his dependence on pain medications would hurt him in many different ways, but for years he continued to take them because he didn't know how else to manage his emotional pain. Despite feeling the sting of what he has lost, Randal remains in control of himself and his life and strives to be the best father possible. His story illustrates an important point: Neither chemical nor emotional addictions define who we really are inside.

Something Else

Nobody wants to be left naked out in the cold. So what special clothes did Randal need to stay warm during his journey? What gives people like Randal the drive to face their addictions and make changes is the *something else.* Those who are dependent on substances can rarely, if ever, just drop the addiction without replacing it with something else. Randal replaced his addiction with firm commitments to his health and children. He certainly needed and received help in the form of education in managing his pain in alternative ways, structured physical rehabilitation, and emotional counseling, all of which were offered in a very secure environment by a nurturing staff. Another important tool was a medication called *buprenorphine,* which I'll explain more about later. It is currently sold in the United States as Suboxone and Subutex. These were all important tools for Randal, but they would have been useless without his commitment.

Doctors have long been taught to use opioids to treat debilitating pain, even when it is more chronic in nature, for these drugs were believed to improve function and quality of life. But over time it's become clear that this approach doesn't provide satisfying long-term results. It may block pain for a while, but it also "blocks" the person and can lead to more pain in the long run. We have also discovered that patients who voluntarily wean themselves off of narcotics seem to do better in general. They are more motivated to go back to work and exercise and generally have better relationships. Of course, weaning oneself off of narcotics can be difficult, if not impossible, for many people. And the relapse rate is usually higher when an addiction is stopped cold turkey.

Not too long ago my partner, John Massey, MD, came across some articles about a medicine called buprenorphine as a treatment for narcotic (opioid) addiction. Buprenorphine binds tightly to the opioid receptors in the brain, preventing narcotics from exerting any effect. This means that when buprenorphine is in your system, other narcotic pain pills will not have any effect on you. In addition, buprenorphine is a partial agonist, meaning it exerts effects of its own. Impressed by what he read, Massey wanted to see if buprenorphine could help a patient named Judy who was in dire straits.

When Judy was in her late twenties, she strained her back and was diagnosed with degenerative disk disease. Her pain was chronic, and she started taking narcotic painkillers daily. Sometime later Judy had a baby. A month after delivery she underwent a three-level fusion surgery (disks in her spine were fused at three different points) because she thought it would help her take better care of her newborn. Unfortunately, Judy felt so miserable after the surgery she could barely get out of bed. She was placed on high dosages of the narcotic drug Oxycontin to help dull her pain so she could walk.

When Massey saw Judy two years later, she was still in terrible pain and taking large dosages of Oxycontin. Her husband had left her, and she was depressed to the point of being suicidal. Massey wanted to enroll her in our comprehensive program, but he was concerned that her excessive use of medication would thwart her success. Because she was so fragile emotionally, he decided to transition her from Oxycontin to buprenorphine at a hospital where she could be monitored closely. He was amazed at how smoothly everything went! Her withdrawal symptoms were fleeting and easy to manage. Her mood perked up quickly, and she became much sharper mentally. Judy left the hospital and began coming to our center, highly motivated to succeed and with enough clarity of mind to learn and process her own emotions.

Today Judy has a new life with a new husband, and owns her own home. She still experiences pain, but is now in charge of her destiny.

Important Facts about Buprenorphine

- It is currently available in the United States only in sublingual form, which means it must be absorbed under the tongue.
- Physicians are required to have a special license to prescribe the drug.
- Common side effects include nausea, constipation, and drowsiness if the dose is too high.

Buprenorphine Plus

Judy's situation improved so rapidly and dramatically that Massey and I began recommending to other patients that they shift from narcotic drugs to buprenorphine. Most of them were very satisfied with the results, feeling they were more in control of what went into their bodies and able to think more clearly.

Once we started to use buprenorphine routinely with opioid-dependent patients, we were amazed at the positive results. We weaned some of our most complicated cases off of their drugs with buprenorphine, then treated them in the supportive environment of our comprehensive program. Tracking their progress, we found that more than 90 percent of these patients were able to stay off their old medications. A full 60 percent went back to work, even though most had been on disability for five years. This was amazing, for statistics show that most people who are on disability longer than six months never return to work. Five years of disability is considered practically hopeless!

Not only that, but after our patients had taken buprenorphine for a few weeks, all kinds of suppressed emotions started to come out. Psychological baggage like anxiety, fear, depression, and past traumas, submerged by addiction-producing medications, suddenly began to make an appearance. One subgroup of patients we see who are prone to addiction are those with a childhood history of attention deficit disorder (ADD) or hyperactivity. For most of their lives, these folks have been medicated by prescription drugs, alcohol, or street drugs in an attempt to quell their racing minds and overactive behavior. Prescription narcotics seem to have a similar effect on them, which means letting go of these medications can unleash a surge of emotions from within that they may not yet be comfortable managing without assistance.

We found that it was extremely important to have our behavioral health staff ready to intervene. For many this means learning to process and cope with internal stressors that have remained latent for many years. In Randal's case, his self-esteem plunged after his very first back injury. The more his back bothered him, the more worthless he felt, and losing some of his sexual function really shattered his sense of self-worth. He used his addiction to painkillers as a way to hide from and numb the hurt. He became addicted to those negative thoughts about himself long before he lost control to Norco. In retrospect I think Randal would agree that it would have been better to work through the self-esteem problem than to lose several years of his life to a medication fog.

Is a "Medicine Shift" Best for You?

We have found that shifting from narcotic drugs to buprenorphine has helped many of our patients, but there are some cases for whom it may not be the best idea, at least not right at that moment. Together you and your physician can determine if and when it's right to wean yourself off narcotic painkillers and start taking buprenorphine instead.

Here are situations that I have found are favorable for making this shift:

- You find yourself requiring more and more pain pills.
- You require extra pills to perform simple activities or fall asleep.
- You run out of your medications before you are supposed to.
- You are spending more time sitting or lying down than before.
- You are having trouble concentrating or learning new information.

Here are a few points to consider *before* doing anything:

- Find out about your options for treatment. Search online and consult with medical professionals who have expertise in pain management, addiction, and buprenorphine treatment. Local hospitals can often provide referral information.
- A strong support team can provide invaluable help in overcoming addictions. Find a comprehensive program staffed with highly qualified, well-trained professionals.

- The insights provided in this chapter are geared toward the treatment of chronic pain that has generated an addiction. The approach to the treatment of primary addictions (like gambling or heroin) falls outside the context of this discussion.

Take the Positive Step!

As you stand at this crossroads, looking to free yourself of your addiction and move toward a healthier and happier life, here are some basic principles worth remembering:

- *Everyone* is afraid of letting go.
- You may not fully appreciate the impact of your addictions until you let go of them.
- Unrecognized addictions can keep you *"stuck,"* and therefore they stand in the way of you taking charge of your life.
- Addictive medications, like narcotics, directly affect the motivational center of your brain, preventing you from doing the things you need to do to move forward.
- Overcoming an addiction requires more than simply changing medications. There must be a comprehensive program in place to support all the physical and mental changes you must make.
- The more tools you develop to manage your pain, the easier it will be to avoid unhealthy habits.
- Not everyone succeeds the first time. Be persistent.

There is something powerful about making a commitment to give up an unhealthy dependency. It is, above all, an act of faith in yourself and what you can accomplish, and most assuredly it is a positive step toward a healthier and happier future.

Even as you work toward ridding your system of harmful chemicals, you still need to nourish your mind and body with health-enhancing substances. In the next chapter we'll look at how to find the foods and nutrients that help the body stave off the harmful effects of chronic pain.

CHAPTER 15

Feed Your Health: Nutrition to Fight Pain

"The doctor of the future will give no medicine, but will interest his patients in the care of the human frame, in diet, and in the cause and prevention of disease."

—Thomas Edison

Food, diets, and eating get more attention in popular culture today than just about any topic imaginable. Bookstores and magazine racks are crowded with publications hawking "magical" foods that can make us look and feel better. Diets, eating plans, and weight-loss strategies abound, but which ones really work? Atkins? *South Beach? Why French Women Don't Get Fat? Skinny Bitch?* And what about eating to ease chronic pain? Is such a thing even possible?

No foods have been proven to directly relieve specific pains, just as there are no foods that cure diseases. But remember: A major focus of this book is to help you become healthier overall, which is key to helping you manage your pain. Experience has taught me that the healthier you become, the less your pain will limit you. A lot of what I discuss in this book doesn't directly alleviate pain, but it can get you to the point—the healthy point—where your pain is ultimately better controlled.

Proper nutrition is one of the most important building blocks of good health. If your nutritional habits are not rock solid, you cannot be 100 percent healthy, no matter what else you do. Working out in the gym four hours every day is great, but if you go home and scarf down a big bag of potato chips and a six-pack of beer, you're undermining your overall health.

That's not to say that there are no links between food and your pain. For example, the stress response and inflammation associated with chronic pain is harmful and painful. An anti-inflammatory diet can help counteract some of these harmful changes and protect the brain and body. Good nutrition helps rebalance the stress-damaged body. And some new research suggests that fish oils containing omega-3 fatty acids and vitamin D have some pain-relieving effects that can be helpful in reducing musculoskeletal pain, the pain of fibromyalgia, and other types of pain problems.

This chapter is about healthful eating in general, for good nutrition is a necessary step in building a healthier you.

The Link between Chronic Pain and Diet

What and how much you eat can affect your pain levels. That's because pain triggers a stress response that produces inflammation, which sets the stage for health problems like heart disease, diabetes, Alzheimer's disease, and in some cases, cancer. (I'm not just talking about the type of inflammation you can see, like a swollen, sprained ankle, but also the silent type that afflicts your heart, brain, and nerves.) Many of these inflammation-driven diseases can increase your pain levels. What you eat can make matters worse, because some foods actually promote the inflammation response, increasing both your pain levels and your chances of developing chronic, debilitating diseases.

Another factor in the food–chronic pain equation is obesity. Obesity is a known risk factor for cardiovascular disease, hypertension, arthritis, certain cancers, diabetes, and other chronic diseases. About one-third of the adult population is obese, while another third is overweight and at risk of becoming obese. One of the "by-products" of pain is inactivity, and in my practice I have found a strong association between obesity and chronic pain. The most obvious link is that excess weight puts pressure on the joints, muscles, and organs and makes it difficult (if not painful) to move the body. This can create a vicious cycle: Pain promotes inactivity, which leads to weight gain, which increases pain. A less obvious problem is the fact that white adipose tissue—the kind that accumulates in the abdomen—produces substances called adipokines, which create inflammation. This is one of the reasons why abdominal fat is considered more dangerous than fat that accumulates elsewhere on the body. For these reasons, keeping body weight down to a moderate level is crucial to controlling or preventing chronic pain.

Luckily there are other foods that do just the opposite and quell inflammation. Not only does food have an impact on how you respond to pain and stress, it can be a deciding factor in the kinds of chronic diseases you develop—or don't develop—along the way.

Let's Go Grocery Shopping

Because poor nutrition can accentuate the inflammation that's already present in injured areas and simultaneously pose added health dangers, it's critical that you carefully choose what you eat. The easiest way to think about the foods that can build and maintain your health and help keep chronic pain levels at a minimum is to visualize the way a grocery store is organized. Typically, the fresher and healthier foods are arranged along the store perimeter. That's where food still looks like food: fruits and vegetables, poultry, fish, meat, and dairy products. In general the more processed and less nutritious foods (like Cap'n Crunch and Doritos) are found in the middle aisles, so be careful when strolling through them!

Pigment Paradise

One of the safest places to choose foods is in the produce section, where the food is unprocessed (it's either pulled out of the soil or plucked off a plant) and contains most of its original nutrients and fiber. Fruits and vegetables are typically high in fiber, low in calories, and chock-full of vitamins and minerals. Which ones are best? Think "rainbow foods"—the more colorful the better. For example, dark green vegetables like spinach, broccoli, and kale are rich in folic acid, beta carotene, and vitamins C, E, and K. Yellow-orange and orange vegetables like squash, carrots, and pumpkin are very high in beta carotene, which has been linked with lower risks of certain cancers and heart disease. Red foods such as tomatoes and watermelon have large amounts of lycopene, which can lower inflammation and dramatically reduce the risk of developing prostate cancer. Blueberries and other purple blue foods contain anthocyanins, which help fight inflammation, strengthen the walls of blood vessels, boost brain function, slow aging, and improve circulation.

All of these rainbow foods are rich in antioxidants, which can help clean up the free radicals thought to be a major cause of disease and aging. They may also help slow the progression of chronic diseases, including those associated with inflammation.

Naturally grown fruits and vegetables have other benefits too: They have a high fiber content, are relatively low in calories compared to other foods, and help balance blood sugars. High-fiber diets help lower cholesterol and lipid levels and keep glucose levels more stable in the blood, but you won't find much fiber in processed, packaged foods. We will soon see why avoiding spikes in blood sugar is so necessary to avoid.

Here are just a few examples of rainbow foods for your shopping list. Pick what you enjoy most, keep an open mind, and don't be afraid to try new things:

- Apples
- Apricots
- Bean sprouts
- Berries (especially blueberries)
- Broccoli
- Brussels sprouts
- Cabbage
- Cantaloupe
- Carrots
- Cauliflower
- Cherries
- Citrus fruits
- Cranberries
- Kale
- Kiwi
- Peaches

- Peppers, green
- Peppers, red
- Pomegranates
- Green vegetables, like spinach
- Tomatoes
- Watermelon
- Winter squash

I prefer fresh foods because they usually taste better, can be eaten raw, and tend to have more nutrients than precooked foods or frozen foods that have to be cooked in order to be eaten. However, frozen foods are reasonable alternatives when fresh foods are not available.

Herbs and spices are also worth mentioning, because many of them— oregano, basil, bay leaves, dill, mint, thyme, parsley, and rosemary—are loaded with nutrients and antioxidants. More exotic choices like cumin, fenugreek, coriander, cinnamon, ginger, and turmeric have been used medicinally in Asian and Indian cultures for centuries. Turmeric, one of the strongest antioxidants in existence, has long been used in India for gastrointestinal ailments, and modern scientists have discovered that it has the potential to reduce inflammation, lower the risk of cancer, improve liver detoxification, protect circulation, and boost brain function in the elderly. Ginger helps treat nausea, improve digestion, lower blood pressure, and reduce plaque build-up in the coronary arteries. It also reduces swelling and inflammation and has a compound that can reduce pain.

Good Fat, Bad Fat

Let's leave produce and move over to the butcher section. The good news is that there is a lot of protein in this section, which is important for building strong muscles and other important body functions. This good news is tempered a bit, however, by the fact that some of the butcher's items also contain a lot of fat, which means you should select wisely to get the best results. I took inventory in a chain grocery store near my house to prepare for this book. It seemed that anything that came in a package in the meat section, whether it was hot dogs, bacon, or turkey, contained the preservative sodium nitrite. If you consume large quantities of processed meats and poultry, be aware that sodium nitrite can be a carcinogenic, and the government regulates its use in foods.

There are some important things to know about dietary fat. First of all, not all fat is bad. In fact, eating the right fats, including essential fatty acids, is a requirement for great health. Essential fatty acids are fats the body and mind need for optimum health but cannot be made by the body; we must get them through food. Nuts and avocados are examples of good sources of essential fatty acids, which are typically unsaturated fats. These fats contain antioxidants and help improve brain and nerve function, strengthen circulation, and fight cancer and heart disease. Eating the right fats actually decreases inflammation and reduces the risk of having a heart attack.

The unhealthy fats are the saturated fats and trans fats. These fats are pro-inflammatory, and will increase cholesterol and promote heart disease. Saturated fats are usually found in fatty animal products like red meats and bacon. Trans fats, which are now considered to be one of the most harmful products in the American diet, are usually found in the processed foods that line those middle aisles of the grocery store. Trans fats may be hydrogenated or partially hydrogenated to give them a more solid consistency, as in margarine. If you read labels, you will find hydrogenated fats in most processed and baked products sold in your local market.

A great source of healthy fat is salmon, as it has an abundance of omega-3 fatty acids. Other fish, including sardines and tuna, also offer high amounts of omega-3 fatty acids, but salmon is best. Be aware of where the salmon you buy comes from, however. Wild salmon is preferable to farm-raised salmon, as it tends to have more omega-3 fatty acids. Fish raised on farms are often fed food that leaves them without the plentiful supplies of omega-3 found in wild fish. What's more, you need to be careful not to eat too much farm-raised fish, as well as too much canned tuna, which may be high in toxins like mercury. Keep in mind, however, that organically farmed salmon may be a reasonable alternative to wild salmon. If you aren't a fan of fish, flaxseed can be an alternative source of omega-3 fatty acids. Nuts, including almonds, walnuts, pecans, and hazelnuts, are also sources of omega-3 fatty acids.

Olive oil is the best all-around oil to use for cooking and seasoning. It has a great track record going back thousands of years and is a key ingredient in the healthy Mediterranean diet, where its consumption is credited with lower rates of cardiovascular disease. Olive oil is a monounsaturated fat with lots of healthy oleic acid, which is an omega-9 fatty acid. Be aware, however, that some manufacturers of olive oil are now mixing in other oils, like peanut oil, to lower costs. Be sure you only buy pure olive oil. Canola oil, also a monounsaturated fat, is an alternative oil to consider.

Not everything in the butcher section is high in saturated fat. Even different cuts of red meat can vary widely in their fat content. Chicken and turkey breasts, sirloin steak, filet mignon, and lamb are some of the butcher items that are relatively low in saturated fat. On the other hand, prime rib, New York strips, rib eyes, and pork chops have some of the highest quantities of saturated fat and so should be eaten in moderation. For example, a sirloin steak has about eighteen grams of fat, with only nine grams of that being saturated fat; a similar size piece of rib eye has double the amount of total fat and saturated fat, plus an extra two hundred calories. As for prime rib, I would save it for really special occasions, as a sixteen-ounce piece packs a whopping ninety-four grams of fat—over half of it saturated fat—and thirteen hundred calories!

Since we're talking about fats, let's head over to the dairy section. Cheese has now become the leading source of saturated fat in the American diet. Cheeses, just like meats, vary quite a bit in their fat content, so read labels. The amount of fat they contain is based on the type of milk used to make them: whole, reduced, nonfat, or cream. For example, because it is made from cream, cream cheese is high in fat. Cheeses made from whole milk include Brie, Swiss, and cheddar; a one-ounce serving of cheddar cheese contains fourteen grams of total fat, compared to half a gram of fat in a four-ounce serving of nonfat cottage cheese. Reduced-fat dairy products also contain lower levels of saturated fats. On the positive side, cheese is typically well stocked with healthier essential fatty acids like conjugated linoleic acid. Low-fat cheeses and unsweetened yogurts can be good sources of protein. Butter is high in saturated fat, but margarine has trans fats, which makes it a poor alternative.

If you like extra flavor in your yogurt, I suggest you add it yourself. All the flavored and sweetened yogurts that I looked at in the market contained something called high fructose corn syrup. Before I explain why you want to avoid that, let me just say that every time I looked at the ingredients of packaged items, they most assuredly had either sodium nitrites, hydrogenated fats, high fructose corn syrup, or some combination of the three.

Avoid the Sweet Spot

Let's move on to the bakery section of the grocery store to learn more about sugars and starches—and high fructose corn syrup. First you need to understand the concept of the *glycemic index,* which measures how quickly certain foods cause a spike in blood sugar (glucose) after they are eaten. This is important, because spikes in blood sugar mimic the body's stress response, which leads to increased inflammation. If the sugar spikes on an ongoing basis, insulin resistance and diabetes can develop, which is like putting the body into a state of chronic stress. And, as you will see in chapter 18, excess glucose in the circulation can build up in the cartilage, leaving the joints stiffer and more painful to move.

Foods that rate high on the glycemic index break down into sugar quickly and overwhelm the body's ability to keep blood sugar levels in balance. Foods that rate lower on the index, such as whole-grain starches and most fruits and vegetables, are digested slower in the intestines, because they have more fiber. This means there isn't a surge of glucose flooding the bloodstream. Comprehensive glycemic index lists can be found in many diet and nutrition books. Be aware of the following commonly eaten foods, which score high:

- White bread and bagels
- White rice and pasta
- Potatoes
- Dried fruit
- Watermelon, corn, and bananas

Because processed and polished starches found in foods like white bread, white rice, and pasta score high on the glycemic index, you want to seek out alternatives that contain whole grains whenever possible, or just eat fewer starchy foods. Substituting fruits, vegetables, nuts, and meats for starchy foods will likely lower stressful sugar spikes in your blood and decrease your daily caloric intake, which will also reduce body fat. Other great starch alternatives that also have bountiful supplies of antioxidants include buckwheat, lentils, barley, and beans. There are times, however, when high glycemic index foods are appropriate to eat. The best time to consume them is around periods of intense physical activity, when exhausted muscles are looking to replenish their sugar supplies.

The glycemic problem runs deeper than just white flour, though. High fructose corn syrup has become the sweetener of choice for most premade foods and soft drinks. Once you head into the middle aisles of the grocery store, where a lot of processed foods like cookies, cereals, and crackers are sold, you will find high fructose corn syrup listed on most of the labels. High fructose corn syrup is corn syrup that is processed to increase its fructose content. A large percentage of this country's calories now comes from this sweetener. The U.S. Department of Agriculture estimates that the average American consumes over sixty-three pounds of it each year. Nutritionists have been concerned for years about the correlation between the jump in the use of high fructose corn syrup and the concurrent increase in the incidence of diabetes and obesity. High fructose corn syrup contains a combination of fructose and glucose, as does table sugar, but it has become such a prevalent sweetener in processed foods because it is cheaper and easier to cook with than table sugar. Unfortunately, foods containing high fructose corn syrup are usually high in calories and carry a high glycemic index.

I almost made the mistake of assuming that my grocery store's in-house bakery would offer healthier alternatives to the items offered in the prepackaged baked goods aisle, but just to be sure, I read through the ingredients of things like sandwich rolls, buns, and pastries. To my surprise, not only was everything baked with high-glycemic refined starches, but partially hydrogenated trans fats and high fructose corn syrup repeatedly popped up on the labels! I could feel my coronary arteries get stiff just sniffing this stuff.

Drink Up

Fluid intake is also a critical part of good nutrition. Our bodies are, after all, mostly water. Decreases in the hydration, or water level, of certain body tissues is associated with certain pain problems and aging. For example, the intervertebral disks in our backs and necks dry up, or dessicate, as you get older. This can lead to degenerative disk disease and spinal stenosis, which can cause back pain and neck pain or sciatica. Well-hydrated disks receive good circulation and look fuller and healthier, just as skin looks younger and suppler when it is well hydrated.

How many glasses of water should you drink each day? Is it eight, as some suggest? It depends on the individual person and what activities he or she does on any particular day. For example, if you go for a strenuous hike or walk one day, you need to drink more water than on a day when you just sit at your desk. A great way to gauge how much water you need is to look at your urine. The darker it is, the more dehydrated you probably are. The clearer it is, the more hydrated your tissues are likely to be. Tap water in certain areas across the country may contain too many toxins, however, so I recommend using a water purifier.

The next great beverage debate concerns coffee. Ever since the Boston Tea Party, America has been infatuated with the coffee bean. Unfortunately, caffeine is a potent diuretic, and too much of it can cause the dehydration that interferes with having a healthy spine and joints and beautiful skin. Caffeine also causes a surge in stress-activated mediators and therefore has pro-inflammatory properties. Then there are those folks who are addicted to those large, supersize "caffeine cocktails" from places like Starbucks, which are also high in sugar and calories. Many feel obliged to drink coffee throughout the day to "keep going," but I consider that a recipe for burnout.

The body's stress hormones, such as cortisol, naturally rise in the early morning; that is thought to be the reason why heart attacks are more common in the morning. Adding a heaping dose of caffeine causes cortisol levels to spike to even higher levels, but many people do it anyway because otherwise they feel too sluggish to attack the day. About three hours after consuming the caffeine, though, their energy starts to wane and they feel taxed again. This can create a vicious cycle that lasts the entire day, forcing them to repeatedly ingest coffee, energy drinks, sodas, or candy for spurts of energy. The resulting highs and lows exhaust the body's circuits, making it even more difficult to get restful sleep. On the flip side, coffee contains its own antioxidants, and some argue that there is some health benefit to a cup of joe.

Green and white teas are another story. I have found these beverages to be vastly superior alternatives to coffee. They are much richer in healthful antioxidants, contain much less caffeine, and have chemicals believed to decrease body fat and improve glucose balance. Darker teas, like black tea, have more caffeine and less antioxidants than green and white tea do. Consider replacing most of your coffee with a few cups of green or white tea per day. My guess is you will feel better as a result. One of the really cool things about drinking tea is that there is a vast variety of flavors to choose from. Even though I started drinking tea about five years ago, I am not even close to running out of new flavors to enjoy.

If you are a big coffee drinker and try to stop, expect to have some frontal headaches for a few days. Rebound headaches from caffeine withdrawal are common. Hang in there, though, because they will eventually go away.

Another beverage often tied to reported health benefits is wine. It is now known that drinking one to two glasses of wine a day is generally associated with good cardiovascular health. Wine is rich in antioxidants, but remember, it also contains sugar and calories, so too much will offset its benefits. If you enjoy wine, I recommend drinking it with or after a meal; drinking it on an empty stomach is more likely to cause a spike in blood sugar.

Soft drinks, on the other hand, offer no value to your health. They come loaded with sugar, score high on the glycemic index, and add unneeded salt to the diet. Diet drinks may introduce nerve-toxic chemicals like aspartame into your body and boost levels of the amino acides glutamate and aspartate around brain cells with heavy use. Pain, stress, and possibly artificial sweeteners can cause excess levels of glutamate and aspartate to float around the brain, and this imbalance can destroy neurons. Recent research shows that drinking diet sodas is actually associated with weight gain, even though they contain almost no calories. One hypothesis is that diet drinks stimulate a hunger for other high-caloric or very sweet foods. I recommend you eliminate soft drinks of all types, and hydrate with purified water and green teas instead.

Kefir, a cultured-milk drink that originated in the Caucus region of Eastern Europe, is considered good for immune system function because it is *probiotic,* or helps increase the levels of beneficial bacteria in the intestines. It differs from yogurt, which is also probiotic, because of the type of bacteria used for the culture. Kefir is high in protein, vitamin D, and calcium and low in saturated fat. While most fruit drinks are too high in sugar to be recommended, mixing a juice rich in antioxidants, like pomegranate juice, with kefir can make a great snack.

Timing Is Everything

Speaking of snacks, many folks equate snacking with poor nutrition and obesity, but it doesn't have to be that way. In fact, eating six small meals per day is associated with less overall caloric intake and better blood sugar balance. For example, having a small snack in the middle of the morning keeps the blood sugar from dipping too low, which allows the body to run more smoothly. Once lunchtime hits, you won't be as hungry so you are less likely to overeat. Frequent smaller meals also lower the strain on the pancreas, which manufactures and releases insulin to control blood sugar levels. If you eat more frequent but small meals, your pancreas won't have to work as hard to keep your sugars in balance.

I recommend you plan your snacks ahead of time and don't leave them up to chance. Avoid the office donuts in favor of foods with a low glycemic index and no trans fats. Something as simple as a handful of almonds offers a great supply of protein and essential fatty acids, with a minimal amount of sugar.

I believe the old adage about breakfast being the most important meal of the day to be true. The time between bedtime and breakfast is the longest period our bodies go without food each day; therefore breakfast is crucial to refueling the body for a productive and efficient day. Studies have shown that folks who regularly eat a substantial breakfast are actually thinner than those who skip breakfast. A hardy morning meal will do a much better job than multiple cups of coffee at keeping your engines humming smoothly, keeping your sugar and cholesterol in balance, and maintaining a slim waist.

The folks on the island of Sardinia, which lies about 120 miles off the Italian peninsula, are considered quite healthy and live longer than people in most other cultures. It turns out that their diets contain high levels of some of the things discussed here. The locally netted sardines are rich in omega-3 fatty acids, and their locally produced wine and sheep's milk cheese are particularly high in antioxidants. They also eat lots of fresh produce, and Italians seem to be quite good at living a low-stress lifestyle.

Eat Mindfully

Now that we have made a round through the grocery store, what do we do with all this information? For recipes and cooking tips, I suggest you consult with some of the famous cookbooks of our time, especially those that have healthful recipes. I would also like you to think about more than just the ingredients you put into your stomach and intestines when you eat. Eating is an experience. Running into the kitchen, throwing a few items into a microwave, then ingesting them while standing up is not what I mean when I talk about an experience. Neither is driving through a fast-food window, grabbing some greasy food, and eating it while driving.

Preparing food for a meal should be much more than a simple, mundane task; it is actually an act of love. Even if you will be the only person eating what you make, you can honor your body and soul by making something special to nourish and please it. The same can be said for others, if the meal is to be shared with friends or family. The meal you create reflects your kindness, generosity, and grace. Take a moment to experience the fragrances and colors of the food. How does it feel when you hold it or taste it? Does the meal you have created bring people together for sharing and laughter? Because meals can be churned out so quickly in our fast-paced world, we run the risk of missing these valuable experiences, which leaves our senses dull.

Let's use our knowledge of nutrition to nourish our body and soul, as well as help prevent the progression of pain and the development of some of our society's most debilitating chronic diseases. The foods we eat directly impact the weight we place on our joints and spines, the strength of our muscles, the amount of inflammation in our bodies, and the health of the blood that travels through the vital organs like our hearts, brains, and livers. Food should never be an afterthought! Instead it should be an ongoing opportunity to cleanse your systems of harmful toxins and inflammation, while taking in plenty of the right nutrients.

These simple steps create an anti-inflammatory diet:

- Eliminate the *white menace:* sugar and foods made of white flour that are quickly converted into sugar. Read labels and watch out for high fructose corn syrup.
- Avoid excessive salt. Premade meals and fast foods are usually pretty salty, so if you avoid them, your salt intake will automatically subside.
- Throw out processed foods. This will help you stay away from trans fats, high fructose corn syrup, and other sources of empty calories.
- Reduce your dependence on caffeine for optimum mental and physical performance.
- Drink clean water.
- Consider switching to organic foods.
- Make foods rich in antioxidants, such as the rainbow foods, the staple of all your meals.
- Eat foods rich in omega-3 fatty acids in place of foods high in saturated fats.
- Don't eat more calories a day than you burn in a day. You can use the Mayo Clinic's Calorie Calculator to get a rough idea of the number of calories you need to burn daily. It's on their Web site at http://mayoclinic.com/health/calorie-calculator/NU00598.
- Don't crash diet! This can cause you to lose important muscle mass and slow down your metabolism. Eat well but smart, and the fat will gradually burn off without destroying the muscles you need to protect your joints and spine.
- Never skip breakfast, and eat about six small meals per day.
- Have some protein with each meal.
- Add the right supplements to your diet to optimize your results.

Supplements

The average American diet has an abundance of calories but is sadly lacking in nutrients. In fact, current estimates hold that 70 percent of Americans are overweight, while 80 percent are malnourished. Besides poor food choices, one reason for this epidemic of malnutrition may be overeating itself. When we overeat, the extra calories add to the workload placed on our mitochondria, the energy generators of the cells. The mitochondria must then work harder to clear the free radicals, toxins, and wastes that are produced from the metabolism of excess calories. Thus chronic overeating overtaxes the system and burns out the mitochondria. Antiaging experts believe that the longer the mitochondria can carry on without burning out, the longer the lifespan. So you may literally be eating yourself into an early grave!

One way to help fight the rampant malnutrition that affects just about everybody is to take supplements. You can think of the typical American body as a car that is burning a lot of gas. It needs additional oil to keep it running smoothly, or the sludge will start to build up and the engine will break down. The "oil" comes in the form of vitamins, minerals, and other supplements.

New research is showing that vitamin D holds promise as a supplement that combats some aches and pains. A deficiency of vitamin D has been linked to chronic pain, including generalized bone and muscle aches. Even though our bodies use sunlight to manufacture vitamin D, deficiency still seems to be widespread. Supplementation of at least 2,000 IU has recently been shown to reduce chronic pain symptoms from problems like arthritis, low back pain, and fibromyalgia. Dairy products and seafood are also good sources of vitamin D.

The following supplements may help optimize your health and reduce the effects of pain and stress:

- *B vitamins*: Critical to fighting cardiovascular disease and atherosclerosis, they also support nerve and brain function and help repair damaged nerves.

- *Carnosine*: This antioxidant supports healing and nerve and immune function. It may also protect against Alzheimer's disease.
- *Alpha lipoic acid*: This potent antioxidant can boost mitochondrial efficiency and improve glucose tolerance.
- *Acetyl-L-carnitine, L-carnitine, and chromium:* These three supplements seem to improve lipid balance, body weight, and brain function.
- *Omega-3 fatty acids:* These aid brain function, decrease inflammation, and improve cardiovascular health. Fish oil, which contains omega-3 fatty acids, may be a safer alternative to anti-inflammatory medications (chapter 21) for problems like arthritis, back pain, and neck pain.
- *Vitamins A, C, and E*: These antioxidants support immunity and fight inflammation.
- *Calcium and Magnesium*: These minerals are vital to nerve, brain, and bone health.
- *Other antioxidants*: CoQ^{10}, DMAE, and the mineral manganese are potent antioxidants that may help fight stress-related inflammation.

A standard multivitamin contains most of these nutrients, but you will probably have to purchase extra supplements to get alpha lipoic acid, L-carnitine, omega-3 fatty acids, and possibly a few other items. Consult with your doctor and/or pharmacist before starting any new supplements. Check the label of your multivitamin carefully to see what it contains. Unfortunately, not all supplements are created equal or can be trusted. Watch out for those made with artificial coloring, flavoring, trans fats, sugars, heavy metals, and other toxins. Brands that have the USP (United States Pharmacopeia) mark are more likely to be of higher quality. USP sets standards for the quality, purity, strength, and consistency of these products. Always check labels or consult with your pharmacist if you are unsure about what you are reading.

Herbs for Chronic Pain

There are thriving cultures today that continue to take advantage of centuries-old remedies to manage health and wellness. For example, millions of people around the world rely on traditional Chinese medicine or ayurvedic medicine from India. Most of the natural tonics used are valued for their abilities to boost overall health, as opposed to being considered disease specific or targeting a certain problem. While they aren't expected to directly reduce pain, integrative medicine specialists like Andrew Weil, MD, recommend them as tools to address some of the secondary effects of chronic pain, like low energy and diminished libido. However, herbal supplements cannot and should not be expected to take the place of good nutrition. Taking fish oil or astragalus isn't going to bail you out if you continue to eat loads of trans fats and high-glycemic foods.

With that in mind, here are a few examples of such remedies:

- *Arctic root:* Originating in the arctic areas of Scandinavia, Siberia, and China, arctic root has antioxidant properties and has been used as a treatment for chronic diseases and infertility and to boost strength.
- *Ashwagandha:* Also known as ayurvedic ginseng, ashwagandha has been used in ayurvedic medicine for over four thousand years to treat inflammatory diseases and tumors and boost male potency.
- *Ginseng:* In traditional Chinese medicine, ginseng root is used to strengthen the immune system, increase vitality, boost resistance to stress-related illnesses, and treat chronic diseases. Its active ingredients, the ginsenosides, have been shown to have anti-inflammatory and antioxidant properties.
- *Astragalus:* A premier herb used in traditional Chinese medicine since the first century B.C., astragalus is used to boost the immune system, fight viral infections, and keep malignant cancer cells from spreading.
- *Cordyceps:* Also known as "winter worm, summer grass," cordyceps begins as a fungus that grows on the backs of

caterpillars and then becomes a tiny mushroom that grows in fields. It has long been used in China and Tibet as a general wellness tonic that increases energy and stimulates the immune system. In recent years it's been claimed that cordyceps can also improve athletic performance.

- *Dong quai:* A member of the carrot family, this Chinese herb contains compounds that exert a mild estrogenic effect, which is why it's used to relieve menstrual cramps and PMS. Dong quai may also help strengthen the actions of the liver and endocrine system and exert a calming effect on the nervous system.

- *Eleuthro:* Commonly known as Siberian ginseng, the root of the eleuthro plant contains steroidal-like compounds called eleutherosides that calm the early stages of the body's stress response. Eleuthro is also used to increase physical performance and help the body adapt more easily to environmental and physiological changes.

- *Maitake:* A Japanese mushroom, maitake is used to boost immunity. Research has shown that substances in the maitake mushroom can activate immume system components called T-cells, shrink certain kinds of tumors, and, in the case of HIV, protect the immune system cells from destruction.

- *Milk thistle:* Found in Europe, milk thistle enhances liver function and the production of new liver cells thanks to its active ingredient, silymarin. It also increases blood levels of glutathione, a powerful antioxidant; quells inflammation; and controls the oxidation that can damage body cells and tissues.

- *Reishi:* This mushroom, which grows on trees and decaying stumps in China, is sometimes used as an immune stimulant by people with HIV or cancer. It appears to prolong the activity of immune system "soldiers" called macrophages. It may also help relieve the fatigue associated with chronic illnesses.

These and other herbal remedies and supplements may be of benefit to some people. However, just because they are "natural" doesn't mean they're safe. Use the same care when taking herbal supplements that you would when taking prescription medications. For safety's sake have your physician review a list of all the supplements that you're currently taking, as supplements can produce dangerous interactions when combined with prescription medications. And always consult with your physician *before* taking anything new.

A Few Last Words

Chronic pain, like other chronic health problems, can disrupt the body's internal operating systems, including hormone balance, neurologic function, and vascular integrity. In other words, it throws the body out of whack. Fortify your body with fresh, whole foods and plenty of water; use supplements judiciously with your physician's supervision; and cut back or eliminate anti-nutrients—white flour, white sugar, trans fats, caffeine, and sodium. By following the recommendations outlined in the anti-inflammatory diet, you can restore equilibrium and bring your body back to a healthier, more efficient state. By feeding yourself with care, you can do much to decrease inflammation, ease your pain, and counteract the changes created by pain.

The next chapter will show you how to put all that good fuel to great use.

CHAPTER 16
Shake Your Groove Thing: Develop Your Exercise Program

Our bodies are designed for movement. Keeping them inactive only makes pain worse, so let's get down to the business of moving. This chapter includes exercises that universally benefit chronic pain sufferers. I have been offering my own rehabilitation and exercise programs to patients since 2001, so I have the benefit of tapping in to years of studying and monitoring what works best. I consulted with my crew of rehabilitation specialists, including Rachel Feinberg and Mai Huong Ho-Tran, who spend hours every day teaching patients with all types of complex problems and injuries how to move and regain the ability to perform meaningful activities. That's why I can confidently say that the exercises I describe in this chapter all come with convincing track records.

These are simple exercises that don't require fancy equipment or expensive health club memberships. They're not designed for rehabilitation from specific injuries, but rather to help you address typical problem areas seen with chronic pain. Where possible I have offered modifications for different levels of fitness. The one basic piece of equipment I recommend you purchase is an exercise ball. They are easy to find and relatively inexpensive. And remember: It's always safest to consult with a physician or physical therapist before trying new exercises or changing your exercise routine.

I can't emphasize enough the importance of coordinating these movements with fluid breathing techniques. The breath work I discussed in chapter 11 should not be limited to just a few minutes of breathing exercises each day. Instead, incorporate effective breathing skills into as much of your day-to-day activities as possible. When doing a stretch, try concentrating on your breathing. Imagine breathing into an area that feels especially tight. As you exhale, feel the tension release from those same muscles. This really works! Avoid clenching up into a death grip when trying to exercise or stretch. The more relaxed your muscles are, the less they will hurt throughout the day.

Exercise #1: Squatting

Moving the body into and out of a squatting position requires the coordinated movement of many different muscle groups, from the core and trunk down into the buttocks and legs. Squatting exercises can improve functional activities like walking and stair climbing. I suggest you do them against a wall.

The first option is to stand with your back, legs, and head against a wall. Your feet should be hip-distance apart. Press your back against the wall and bend your knees as you slowly and carefully lower yourself into a sitting position. See if you can slide down far enough so that you're sitting in an imaginary chair. Over time slowly try to increase the length of time you can hold this position.

You can add motion to the exercise by propping an exercise ball between your back and the wall. While leaning back against the ball, slowly bend your knees and lower into a squatting position. Then push yourself back up by straightening your legs for one set. Repeat as tolerated.

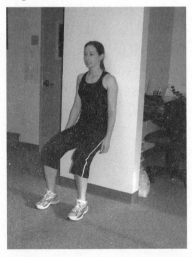 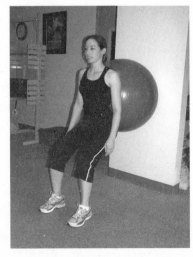

Exercise #2: Bridging

This exercise also engages many important muscle groups around the core and legs. Start off lying flat on your back on the floor. Bend your knees so that your heels move toward your buttocks, then plant your feet on the ground. When your knees are fully bent, raise your buttocks off the ground, keeping your thighs firmly rotating toward each other. Use your hands for support. As you progress, you can start to roll your spine off the floor, too, and then gently roll back down, starting with the top of the back and progressing until the buttock is resting on the floor. Repeat this exercise as tolerated.

A variation is to place your feet on an exercise ball, instead of the floor, while you bridge. An advanced version of bridging includes straightening one leg at a time and raising it off the floor while supporting yourself with the other foot firmly planted.

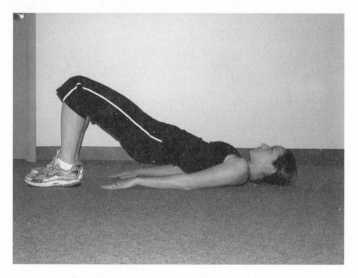

Exercise #3: Reverse Bridge with a Ball

Lie with your back on an exercise ball, maintaining contact between the ball and your lower back. Support your head with your hands, keep your knees bent, and your feet firmly planted on the ground. Roll over the ball with your back until the upper back is resting on the ball and your lower back is supported by your core and legs. Repeat up and down the spine as tolerated.

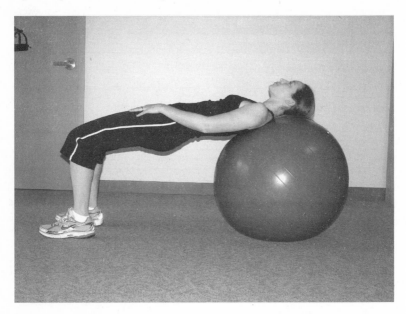

Exercise #4: Plank

The whole body has to work to perform plank exercises properly. Start by lying face down on the floor, resting your forearms on an exercise ball in a secure position. (This will hold your upper back and head off the floor.) Straighten the rest of your body so that only the balls of your feet and toes are touching the floor. Feel your heels push backward while your core and pelvis engage to keep your body lifted. Your body should form a fairly straight line.

A more challenging version of the plank can be performed without the exercise ball. Lie face down on the floor, resting your forearms on the floor, shoulder-width apart and elbows bent at 90 degrees. Your upper back and head should be lifted into the air. Straighten your legs and come up on your toes. Hold this position as long as you can. For an even greater challenge, get into the plank position and then alternate lifting one leg up a few inches off the ground. You can also go into a plank with your arms straight (push-up position) and maintain that position for a few breaths.

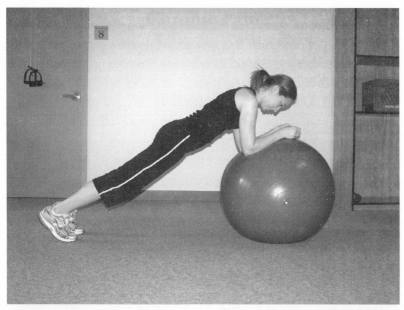

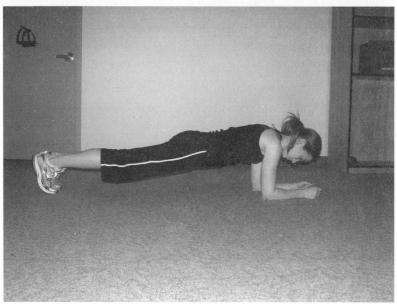

Exercise #5: Child's Pose or Prayer Stretch

You might be thinking that you need a break about now. This pose is a great way to relax for a minute or two and get reenergized. Kneel down on the floor with your knees spread apart and feet touching. Sit back toward your heels; you can go as far as having your buttocks possibly resting lightly on your heels. Stretch your arms out in front of you on the floor, with the palms and fingers on the ground. Your forehead can rest on the floor. Look straight down. Breathe slowly in and out through your nose while your body gently lengthens and relaxes. Try not to let the chest collapse.

For a variation that can be easier on the upper extremities and shoulders, simply rest the arms facing backward next to your legs.

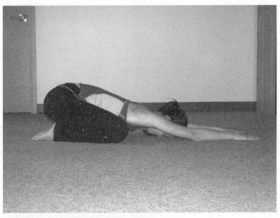

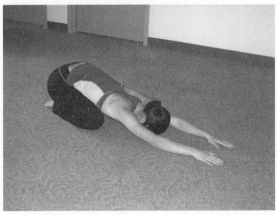

Exercise #6: Push-ups

Push-ups can strengthen a whole lot more than just your chest muscles. They can improve total upper body strength and engage the core muscles. Wall push-ups can be a good place to start. Stand facing a wall; stretch your arms out in front of you, hands on the wall. Bend the elbows as your chest moves toward the wall, then straighten the arms to push the chest away from the wall. Do as many repetitions as you comfortably can. As you progress, you can lower the incline by leaning against something like the back of a couch instead of a wall. This will require added upper body strength.

Push-ups done on the floor are more difficult. One variation is to place the knees on the floor for added support. Keeping your hands planted on the floor, in line with your shoulders, and holding your elbows at your side while they bend and lower you to the floor will work more of your upper body muscles and core. For more challenge, raise the knees up off the floor into a plank position, lower yourself down to the floor, then push up. As your strength builds, you will be able to do more repetitions.

For extra support, try lying face down over an exercise ball at your belt line or your thighs and practice doing push-ups from that position.

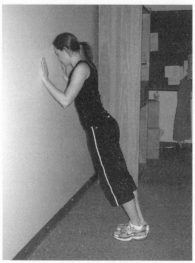

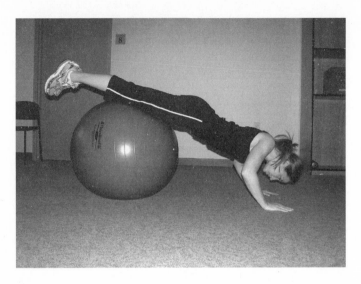

Exercise #7: Dead Bug

There are several variations to this core- and trunk-stabilizing exercise, so start with the beginner's version and work from there. Begin by laying with your back flat on the floor. Your lower back should be firmly touching the floor at all times. It might help if you imagine your belly button pressing your low back down against the ground. Bend the knees, keeping the soles of both feet on the floor. Keeping your left foot on the floor, raise your right knee up so that your right thigh is perpendicular to the floor, and then lower it back down. Now do the same motion with the left leg, while the right foot stays on the floor. Do as many repetitions as you can.

The next step is to start with both knees bent, feet elevated off the ground, and thighs perpendicular to the floor. From this starting position, lower your right foot to the floor while keeping the right knee bent, and then raise it back up, keeping your lower back pressed to the floor. Now do the same with your left foot. That completes one set. Do as many as you comfortably can. Once this gets easy, you can start to use the arms. Begin by raising them straight up in the air. As the *left* leg is dipped to the floor, the *right* arm rotates at the shoulder and is lowered toward the floor (as if you were in class raising your hand). When the left leg comes back up, so does the right arm. Repeat with the opposite legs and arms.

The hardest version of Dead Bug starts with both arms and legs lifted straight up, at a 90-degree angle to the floor, while you are on your back. While keeping the arms and legs straight, and the back pressed against the floor, lower the right arm back overhead toward the floor while simultaneously lowering the opposite left leg down. With control, bring the arm and leg back up to the starting position and repeat with the opposite arm and leg. Make sure that a physical therapist or exercise trainer supervises you when trying this version for the first time.

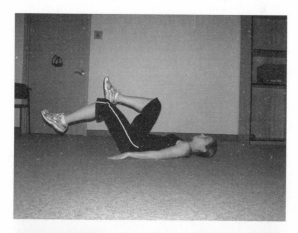

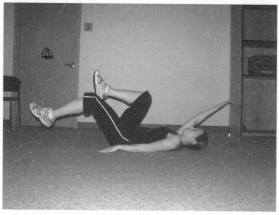

Exercise #8: Hip Flexor Stretch

There are many different ways to stretch the hip flexor muscles. The main muscle of this area is the *iliopsoas,* a large muscle that attaches at the lower back and travels through the pelvis to connect to the thigh. Contracting the iliopsoas pulls the thigh up and raises the leg, which is necessary for activities like walking, cycling, running, or climbing stairs. I have found the iliopsoas muscle to be an unrecognized source of low-back pain in many patients. It often gets tight and rigid, especially with prolonged sitting or after back surgery, which if not treated can limit flexibility, movement, and simple activities.

A simple stretch for the iliopsoas muscle is to assume a lunge position, with the front leg bent at the knee, the back leg stretched behind you, and the back knee touching the floor. Both hands can rest on your front thigh or on the ground next to your front foot. As you gently lean forward toward the front knee, you should feel a stretch on the top of your back thigh. Hold this for thirty to ninety seconds and then reverse legs.

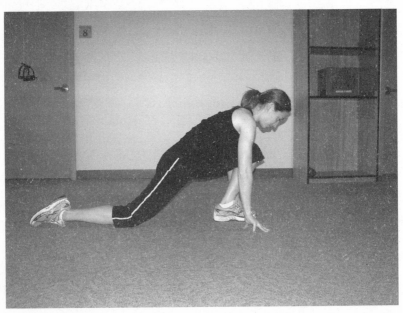

If you have access to a bed or table that rises to about three feet above the ground, try laying face up on it, with your right hip and shoulder perched at the edge. Flex your left thigh toward your chest and hold it with your left hand. Next let your right leg lower off the bed toward the floor. For more of a stretch, hold the right foot with your right hand and gently pull it further and hold. Don't forget to breathe! Change sides to repeat with the opposite leg.

Exercise # 9: Hip Opener

The pelvis and lower back have many other muscle groups that can easily tighten up and cause pain in response to injuries to the knees, hips, and spine. Exercises or stretches designed to lengthen and loosen these muscle groups are sometimes referred to as hip openers. Keeping these hip-opening muscles flexible and developed can help prevent excess wear and tear on joints in the hips, sacroiliac (where the tailbone connects to the pelvis), and lower back.

One particular muscle in the buttock that connects the tailbone to the upper thigh, known as the *piriformis,* helps rotate the thigh away from the body. The piriformis is often specifically addressed by physical therapists and orthopedists because it sometimes wraps around the sciatic nerve. The sciatic nerve is the largest nerve in the body; it travels from the spine down the back of the leg. When the piriformis muscle is suspected of causing sciatic nerve pain to shoot down the back of the leg, the condition is referred to as *piriformis syndrome.*

There are several great yoga poses that help stretch muscles like the piriformis to create more of an opening in the hips and pelvis. A nice one to start with begins with you lying on the floor with your knees bent and legs lifted. Hold your left thigh at a ninety-degree angle to the floor and bend your lower leg to make a right angle with the thigh. Next rotate your right leg up and around until you can rest your right foot on top of your left thigh. The right foot should stay flexed and point up to the sky. This will stretch your right piriformis muscle. Flexing your left thigh toward you will increase the stretch on the piriformis. To increase the stretch, wrap your hands around the back of your left thigh and pull it toward you. After holding for thirty to ninety seconds, switch legs and repeat.

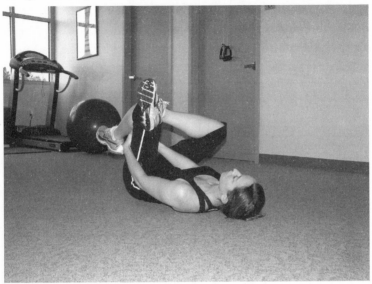

One of my patients, who had suffered from low back pain for several years, recently told me that she had always underestimated the value of stretching in managing her chronic pain until we convinced her to perform this hip opener exercise on a daily basis. This simple stretch helped diminish her daily back pain and became a helpful tool for calming her flare-ups. One lesson she learned is that for a long time she had been unconsciously tightening the muscles around her hips and pelvis as a way to protect her back from further damage, but this was actually causing more discomfort.

Exercise #10: Walking

Because of the evolution in lifestyle habits that has encouraged most of us to spend a lot of our time sitting and very little exercising, walking is a critical member of my exercise to-do list. I will talk more later about the importance of walking to staying young and vibrant, but it is worth noting here that most of us don't walk nearly enough, thanks to phenomenal technological advances in communication and transportation that have occurred over the past fifty or so years. For thousands of years walking was integral to existence. Today many of us can go days at a time without walking farther than from our cars to our houses.

Folks who walk regularly are typically healthier than their more sedentary counterparts. They are less likely to suffer from type 2 diabetes, high blood pressure, heart attacks, obesity, age-related cognitive decline, osteoporosis, and depression. Walking can boost metabolism and burn an extra 100 to 150 calories each hour. For those whose activities are limited by pain, walking may be the best-tolerated way to get aerobic exercise. Just being outside offers benefits like an enhanced mood, more social interactions (which means more chances to smile!), and even improved vitamin D production. This is important, as vitamin D deficiency is on the rise and has been found to be a risk factor for chronic pain.

We have known for many years now that bed rest actually makes back pain worse, while research suggests that walking can be an effective way to reduce low back pain. For example, one study published in 2005 in the *American Journal of Public Health* followed several hundred patients with low back pain and found that those who walked three hours a week had less back pain than those who did specific low back exercises.[15] In general, a stronger body will experience less pain than a weaker one. Consider all the muscles that walking can strengthen, including those in the feet, calves, thighs, buttocks, and trunk, not to mention the heart, and it starts to make sense. Walking also improves circulation to the spine, which will help eliminate toxins and inflammatory mediators. By pulling us up out of our couches and chairs, walking can improve our posture and boost bone density, too.

---

15   Hurwitz, et al. "Effects of Recreational Physical Activity and Back Exercises on Low Back Pain and Psychological Distress: Findings from the UCLA Low Back Pain Study," *Am. J. Public Health.* 2005 October; 95(10): 1825–1831.

The right number of steps, blocks, miles, or minutes to walk depends on the individual. Even if your starting distance is a block or less, it is still better than nothing at all. If you stick with it, there is a good chance that over time you'll be able to cover more and more ground. Remember: You started walking as an infant with just a couple of steps, but in no time at all your parents were chasing you all over the place.

Helpful Hints to Get Started

There are hundreds more exercises that can be useful to build strength throughout the body, increase flexibility, and ultimately reduce pain, than those presented here. These are the top ten that have been found to be consistently and universally beneficial. I suggest you use them as a starting point and build from there. You can continue to add new exercises and movements taught to you by physical therapists, occupational therapists, and exercise instructors. One word of caution: It has been our experience that most of these teachers don't have special training for the highly complex world of chronic pain. They are often more comfortable working with acute sports injuries. If you've had a bad experience where physical therapy seemed to "make it worse," don't give up on finding safe and effective activities you can do to improve your health and reduce your pain.

Here are some pearls of wisdom from my rehabilitation specialists:

- Slow progress is good progress, so be proud of it.
- Start at a point with an activity or exercise that you feel comfortable with and progress from there.
- The more independent you get, the more self-confident you become.
- Understand the difference between acute pain and chronic pain. Sore muscles will quickly feel better.
- You may actually already be doing things that you think you can't. For example, look at all the activity and movement that goes into just getting out of bed.

- Everyone struggles with bending and squatting. You can become a lot more active if you learn how to do these movements using good body mechanics.
- Always practice a movement in a relaxed state and BREATHE. People have a tendency to tense up when doing a challenging activity; this might aggravate your pain.
- Start your stretches GENTLY. Avoid the "pull and yank" approach. Remember: Muscles are fibers.
- The stronger you become, the more confident you will feel.
- If possible, try to understand your anatomy and ignore misguided phrases from your practitioners and friends. Disks don't just "slip" out in your back.

The results my patients get with basic exercises like these are consistently amazing. With eight weeks of structured exercise and activity for two hours a day, I routinely see bodies transform before my very eyes. Some come in using canes and wheelchairs and leave walking on their own accord for the first time in months or even years.

When I first met Anna, for example, she had been suffering for many years from chronic back pain that radiated down her left leg, even after undergoing spine surgery and trying so many strong pain medicines that she couldn't remember all their names. As a child and young woman, she had been very athletic and loved jazz dancing and playing sports, but now she associated movement with pain and so did as little as possible. For Anna, this meant living without many of the things she loved doing, like dancing and playing catch with her kids. However, by consistently performing the exercises above, she was able to find her inner "girl" once again, and movement became fun for her again, including running for the first time since she had first hurt her back.

Because the whole body is affected by an injury in just one of its parts, Anna learned the value of using many different types of exercises to help regain lost function from a specific injury. One of the things I like about these top ten exercises is that, when done properly, they engage different parts of the body, as opposed to isolating one muscle or movement. As we learned in chapter 9, our bodies are happiest when we allow them to move.

More helpful options for movement will come your way in chapter 17, when we look at some very valuable alternative healing practices from across the globe.

Eastern Moves for the Western Soul

Leaving behind the sick role and assuming a wellness-oriented role is a fundamental shift in thinking that I try to help my patients achieve. Traditional Western medicine is geared to help us when we don't feel well; it's a reaction to illness. Although it does emphasize preventive care like Pap smears, mammograms, and colonoscopies beginning at age fifty (I can't wait!), these measures still focus on disease. Their purpose is simply to detect sickness earlier so it can be treated more effectively. While modern medicine provides us with powerful tools to treat many specific diseases, what happens if you have a chronic health problem that isn't a specific disease, is too complicated to eliminate with just a few easy treatments, but makes you feel lousy every day?

If you have chronic pain, this Western "treat the disease" model puts you in the role of a patient each and every day. That can mean doctor appointments for more tests or treatments, visits to the physical therapist, and taking pills every day to treat the effects of being ill. I'm amazed at how many new patient questionnaires I read that describe a typical day as, "Take pain pills to get out of bed and go to doctor appointments." Once you adopt this mind-set, taking pills and going in for more exams and treatments can feel as routine as drinking that morning cup of coffee!

How can you expect to get pleasure from life and feel good about yourself if you believe that you are incessantly ill? How can you possibly enjoy your day if you know that you will be a *patient* for every one of the next twenty-four hours? I've found that it's very important to change the perceived role from being a patient to being a health manager. This means that instead of thinking of yourself as being sick, you think about creating health and wellness for yourself. This is a key concept, for transforming your thought process is the first step toward changing your behavior patterns for the better.

Like most of you, I was raised in the traditional Western medicine milieu, where I only saw my pediatrician when I had a sore lump in the back of my throat, was roasting with a 103°F fever, or was hurling my food across the room at my parents. Most of my medical education took place inside hospitals or within one block of them. There I learned how to treat illnesses and diseases, like infections, heart failure, or massive blood loss from trauma. Nobody ever taught me how to be healthy, let alone create great health for others.

How can we learn to think of ourselves as being well in a system that encourages the opposite? For many the answer lies in looking to the East.

Travel the Silk Road

When I offer my patients suggestions on how to deal with their most pressing needs, I tell them that it would be very helpful for them to

- Manage or decrease **stress.**
- Find **balance** despite a hectic lifestyle.
- Eliminate negative **emotions** and thoughts.
- Become more **active** without increasing pain.
- **Sleep** more restfully.
- Reconnect **relationships** with friends and family.
- **Think** more clearly.
- Improve **circulation** to areas damaged by inflammation or injury.
- Enjoy a more active **sex** life.
- **Learn acceptance.**

Amazingly, Eastern health and medicine philosophies focus on precisely these items. Some of these ancient Chinese and East Asian practices go back over five thousand years, so they have pretty impressive track records.

In the Eastern tradition there is no separation of mind, body, and spirit; they are considered totally integrated. The whole is always more important than the parts. When one part of the body is injured, imbalance is created everywhere and the whole person becomes weak. I love this emphasis on the totality of the person that, when translated into Western medicine-speak, means that when, say, the lower back is hurt, the whole person is affected, body *and* mind *and* spirit.

In traditional Chinese medicine, illness is believed to stem from the blockage of energy *(chi)* to the affected area of the body. It's much like what happens in the case of a stroke. When blood flow to a certain area of the brain is blocked by a blood clot, the brain cells that are "downstream" from the blockage die from a lack of nutrients. The difference between chi and the bloodstream is that chi is invisible and believed to flow through the body along invisible channels called meridians. According to traditional Chinese medicine theory, twelve major meridians run through the body, delivering energy and sustenance to the tissues. If a blockage of chi occurs at any point, pain and disease result. And, again, since there is no separation of body, mind, or spirit in the Eastern tradition, when one area of the body is injured, imbalance is created everywhere and the whole person suffers.

While this may sound very different from the way Western medicine operates, the two aren't so far apart in certain ways. For example, according to Western philosophy, if you avoid using your foot for a full year because it hurts, the muscles will weaken and atrophy and less blood will flow to the area. Similarly, in Eastern philosophy, a blockage keeps the chi from flowing freely through the foot. In order for the foot to heal, the circulation of blood or chi must be restored. But whether you subscribe to the Eastern or Western way of looking at the problem, the foot won't get better until it's being used regularly. Only then will the muscles get stronger, the circulation improve, and the energy increase.

A notable difference in the Eastern and Western approaches to healing concerns the relationship of emotions to illness. In Western medicine illness/injury is thought to cause negative emotions. In other words, having a sore back can make you cranky, while chronic knee pain can make you depressed. In Eastern medicine, however, it's just the opposite: Negative emotions are thought to contribute to chronic disease. The negative emotions don't create the original injury, but they can turn it into something more lingering and disastrous. Taking this a step further, if every emotion is preceded by a thought, as we are taught in modern psychology, then our Asian counterparts would suggest that changing dysfunctional thoughts is the first step to fighting or preventing chronic pain.

A behavioral trait that is particularly likely to bring on chronic pain is *catastrophizing*—believing that something is much worse than it really is. For example, if you're absolutely sure that your wrenched knee will keep you from ever climbing stairs again, you'll probably feel the pain for a much longer period of time. Research has shown that those who catastrophized after straining their backs suffered much more disability than those who were less worried about their injuries. In Chinese medicine, catastrophizing is believed to create imbalances that lead to stress.

The teachings of Buddha also hold some interesting ideas about pain. In Western culture, pain is associated with the presence of disease; its existence implies that you are ill. However, Buddha viewed pain as an unavoidable part of life and something that has to be accepted. He believed that we can learn from our pain if we acknowledge it as an object that is present, and he preached exercising patience when coping with pain. Viewing pain as an object means that you know the pain is there, but you don't develop an opinion about it that alters how you feel inside. If my California brain is interpreting this correctly, he is saying that you must recognize your pain as *pain,* as opposed to viewing yourself as *in pain,* which would then make it a part of your identity. He would probably reject our habit of identifying ourselves according to the names we have given chronic pain diseases, like fibromyalgia or sciatica, out of concern that those terms would become part of who we are.

Instead he would urge us to accept that those problems exist and accept them as part of being alive. And if you can smile about them, even better.

Speaking of smiling, in Eastern philosophy smiling is thought to move the chi to places that are under stress, restore balance, and dissolve negative emotions. It's also believed to feed the thymus gland, which is considered a center of love and enlightenment. Modern medicine recognizes the thymus gland as an integral part of the immune system, making it helpful in fighting diseases like cancer. This seems to dovetail nicely with the old adage that "laughter is the best medicine."

An Eastern Approach to Pain Relief: Exercise Like a Rock Star

Buddhism and other Eastern philosophies infuse Eastern healing traditions such as traditional Chinese medicine, which emphasizes viewing body, mind, and spirit as a single unity and promoting health rather than waiting to treat disease. I'm not a guru in Eastern medicine, but I stumbled across these philosophies of health and believe they hold the key to what's missing in our Western lifestyle and ways of treating disease. A number of the complementary health practices sprouting up all over the United States have roots in the Eastern approach to health. Perhaps Madonna can be credited with making yoga part of mainstream American culture!

As part of our center's comprehensive program, we offer classes in three Eastern practices: qigong, tai chi, and yoga. Practicing any or all three disciplines can help people manage their pain in ways that modern medicine simply can't. Instead of focusing solely on specific body parts that are painful, qigong, tai chi, and yoga connect the mind and body by controlling the body's energy flow. This leads to greater energy, deeper relaxation, improved health, and increased self-awareness. For some this awareness can help relieve certain symptoms. For example, if you tense your shoulders in response to pain, your neck and shoulder muscles may get tight and start to hurt. Once you realize you're doing this, you can consciously change this habit and eliminate that source of pain.

My goal with this chapter is to provide you with basic background training in some of these alternative healing practices. Hopefully this will jump-start your interest in utilizing the resources that may be available in your community. You can probably find classes at gyms, health clubs, community centers, community colleges, and private studios.

So let's take a look at these movement disciplines and see how they work to improve inner balance and health.

Qigong

Qigong is an ancient Chinese medicine practice that coordinates breathing, gentle movement, and meditation to strengthen, circulate, and cleanse the life energy, or *qi*, which is the same thing as chi. In qigong the breath is used to increase the circulation of energy through various exercises. *Qi* means "air" or "life force," and *gong* means "work applied to a discipline." So *qigong* literally means "the practice of breathing."

Qigong is not only invigorating, it is relaxing. The diaphragmatic breathing at the core of the practice is an important part of the relaxation response, and its gentle exercises are calming. Practitioners of qigong learn to control their reactions to stress, thereby reducing the risk of developing stress-related symptoms like pain, high blood pressure, anxiety, depression, and gastrointestinal symptoms. Qigong has been shown to improve posture, increase range of motion, improve joint flexibility and resilience, cause favorable changes in blood chemistry, increase self-awareness, and improve concentration. Research suggests that it may also be beneficial for a wide variety of ailments including asthma, arthritis, cardiovascular disease, chronic fatigue, fibromyalgia, headaches, and pain in general.

Tai Chi

Tai chi originated in China around the thirteenth century as a combination of martial arts and meditation. It was originally developed by Chinese martial arts experts to advance their skills, but it has since been embraced as an effective way to relieve stress and promote health and longevity. Tai chi has been shown to reduce stress, enhance immune function, lower blood pressure, ease anxiety, improve posture and balance, and reduce falls. The increase in the awareness of and ability to maintain balance is important. As we get older, our ability to balance declines if we don't do specific exercises to maintain it. Falls due to poor balance often lead to injuries among the elderly, including broken hips, compression fractures in the spine, and broken ribs. Besides improved balance, tai chi promotes increased range of motion in joints and muscles and better circulation.

Tai chi had a profound effect on Kim's life. Kim had worked as a grocery store clerk for many years, and her duties required continuous lifting and carrying. By the time she reached her forties, she had developed increasing pain in her left hand that began to move up her arm and into her shoulder. What began as an annoying twinge grew progressively worse, until Kim was unable to raise her left arm over her head without it going numb and could no longer lift or carry more than two pounds. As if the pain and disability were not enough, the skin on Kim's left arm started to change; it looked waxy, mottled, and discolored, and her fingers tingled—typical symptoms of a challenging and perplexing problem known as complex regional pain syndrome (CRPS).

Kim's doctors finally told her there was nothing more they could do to help her, but she was determined to not give up and eventually came to our clinic. One of our instructors spent a great deal of time doing tai chi with her, and this enabled Kim to move her injured arm in ways that previously seemed impossible. After several weeks of using tai chi with other treatments, Kim was able to lift twelve pounds with her left arm and safely carry eight pounds.

Her skin coloration and circulation improved, and there was much less numbness when she raised her left arm. Tai chi has now become a daily practice for Kim to maintain her healthy changes and keep her arm functional.

Here are a few examples of tai chi exercises:

- *Tai Chi Posture:* Body is upright but relaxed, head erect, chin slightly pulled in, shoulders balanced and relaxed and aligned over the hips. Pelvis is tilted slightly forward so the rear end can be rolled under a bit. Weight is evenly distributed on the soles of the feet, and arms hang loosely at the sides. When moving, one foot is firmly planted while the other one lifts. Through it all the body remains in an upright position and the shoulders stay aligned over the hips.
- *Opening Stance:* Stand in the tai chi posture with your feet shoulder-width apart. Hang arms loosely at your sides.

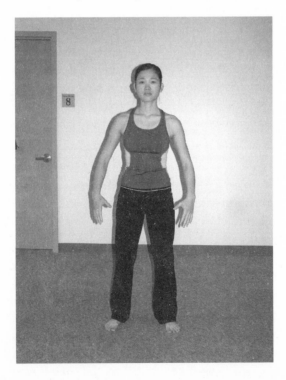

- *Bow Stance:* From Opening Stance, move your left leg forward with your feet shoulder-width apart and toes pointing slightly out. Bend your left knee and shift your weight partially forward. This can also be done with the right leg forward.

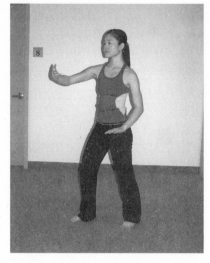

- *Empty Step:* This is a basic tai chi step, where all of your weight is placed on one leg. The other leg grazes the ground but doesn't bear weight.

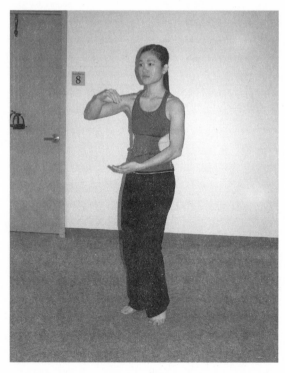

- *Tai Chi Hands:* Your eyes typically follow your leading hand. Your hands should be open in a relaxed manner so as not to block the flow of energy with too much tension. A slight curve in the fingers is recommended.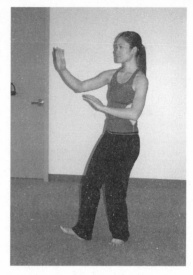

- *Neck Warm-Up:* Start in Opening Stance and let the head gently roll forward, bringing the chin toward the chest. Gradually lift the head until you are looking upward, if possible. This movement can be repeated several times.

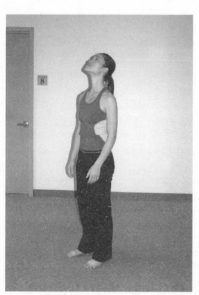 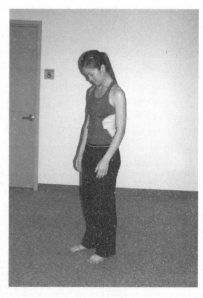

- *Shoulder Exercise:* From Opening Stance, move the fingertips to the tops of the shoulders. Rotate the elbows in wide circles. Repeat in the opposite direction.

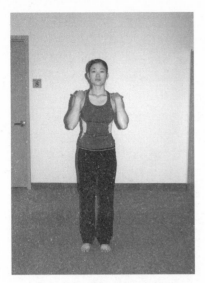 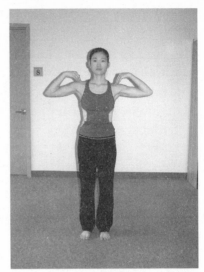

- *Hip Exercise:* Stand erect with hands clasped behind the back or at your sides for balance. Raise the right knee until the thigh makes a ninety-degree angle to the standing leg. Rotate the leg to the right as far as possible. Gently lower the right leg until the ball of the foot touches the ground, but keep the weight on the left leg. Repeat this a few times before switching legs.

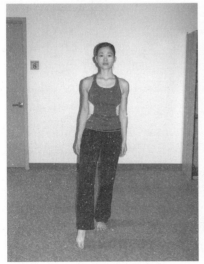 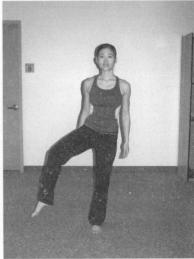

- *Parting of the Clouds:* From Opening Stance, shift to Bow Stance with your left leg forward. Bring your hands together at the waist with the palms facing each other but not quite touching. Shift forward, with your hands reaching in front of you during exhalation. Once they are extended, rotate the palms down. Shift back while inhaling and rotating the arms in a wide circle to the starting position. After doing this several times with the left foot forward, do the same with the right foot forward.

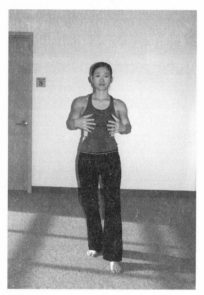 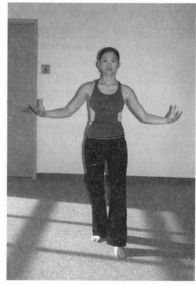

Yoga

Exercise styles and health programs may come and go, but the practice of yoga has survived the test of time. Yoga originated in northern India more than three thousand years ago, but the Western world didn't begin to embrace it until the 1970s. The word *yoga* is Sanskrit for "union" and refers to the union of body, mind, and spirit. The main goals of yoga are to control the mind, body, and breath while connecting to one's spirituality. The practice of yoga involves a series of specific poses, or *asanas,* that are performed while controlling the breath.

Yoga offers many health benefits, including stress relief; improved strength, flexibility, and posture; and better concentration and mental focus. It helps alleviate pain by bringing the body into balance, building strength, increasing flexibility, releasing tension, and strengthening joints and bones. The benefits of yoga are psychological as well as physical. The mind finds a positive focus, instead of focusing on the pain. Deep breathing also helps calm the body and increase relaxation, which can result in a decrease in pain.

The *Sun Salutation* is a well-known sequence of basic yoga positions that aids in pain management by connecting the mind, body, and breath with fluid movements. The Sun Salutation has numerous other health benefits, including greater spine and joint flexibility. There are different versions of the Sun Salutation, one of which goes like this:

1. Stand tall, inhale, and bring your arms overhead.
2. Exhale as you fold forward toward your toes.
3. Inhale as you raise your spine and look forward with your hands on your shins.
4. Exhale as you step or jump your feet back behind you into a push-up position. Lower down to the floor.
5. Curl your spine up off the mat during inspiration, with your shoulders pulled back and hands propping up your torso.
6. Exhale while pushing your hips up and back, with feet firmly rooted on the floor. Gaze at your navel. (This position is commonly known as Downward Dog.)
7. Inhale while you jump or walk your feet forward, and again lengthen the spine forward and up so you are looking straight ahead.
8. Exhale into a forward fold, looking at your toes.
9. Inhale while you rise up to a standing position with your arms raised overhead, palms touching.
10. Exhale while lowering your arms to your sides, ready to repeat.

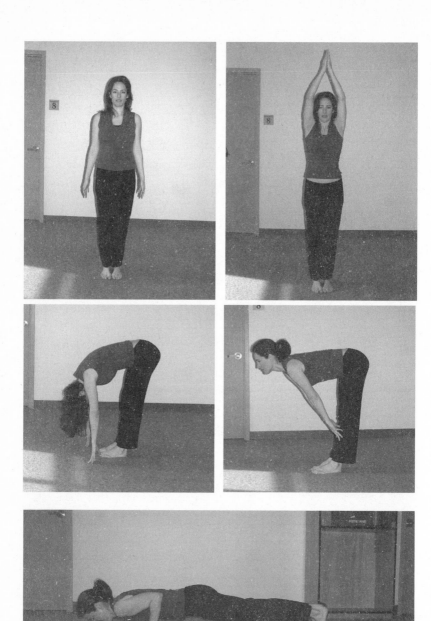

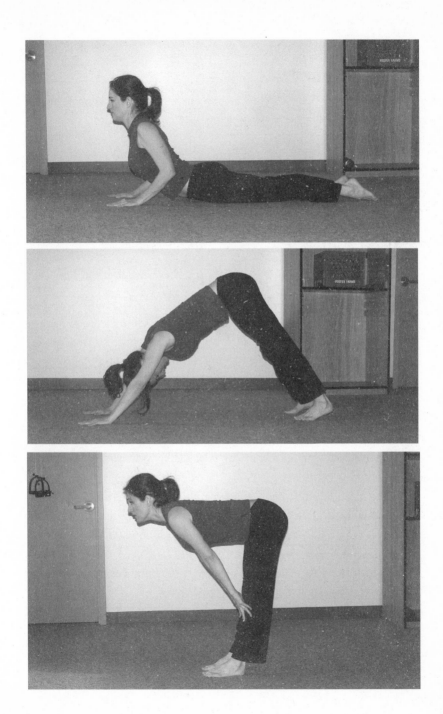

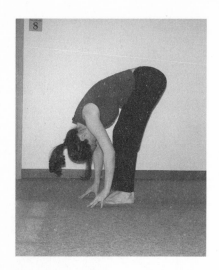
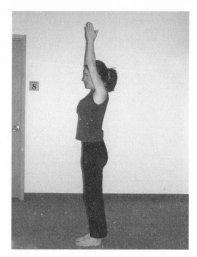

A Western Approach: Pilates

Although Pilates doesn't come from India or China, like the Eastern disciplines it honors the mind/body connection by incorporating unique movements with coordinated breathing. Joseph Pilates, a native of Germany who had moved to England, started his unique brand of exercise during World War I when he was interred with other German nationals. During this time, Joe learned how to rig springs to hospital beds to create exercise equipment that allowed him to work with bedridden patients. After his release he went back to Germany and worked with members of the dance community. Later he immigrated to the United States, where his methods became an integral part of the New York dance community, by rehabilitating injured dancers much more quickly than standard approaches. Joe had a background in self-defense and also trained a number of boxers.

Pilates involves integrated movements of the limbs and trunk, rather than isolated muscle groups. The discipline focuses on posture; breath; abdominal strength; spine, pelvis, and shoulder stabilization; muscular flexibility; joint mobility; and strengthening. It has been shown to be effective in easing low back pain, reducing the need for back surgery and increasing bone density. It's perfect for people as they get older, when they have aches and pains and can no longer play racquetball or engage in other rough-and-tumble activities. As far as I'm concerned, every senior center and retirement community should have Pilates classes or instructors. It's a great way to improve flexibility, range of motion, strength, coordination, and balance, which makes it the perfect anti-aging exercise. It is also excellent as a method of rehabilitation for people who have hurt their backs or other parts of their bodies and still have pain-control issues, and it is an ideal post-rehabilitation form of exercise.

When my patients have spine problems, I often recommend they see a Pilates-trained physical therapist to learn important fundamentals about posture and movement. Once they have the basics down, it may be safe to work with a trainer or take group classes.

Some Pilates instructors are better trained than others, but it can be hard for a beginner to know the difference. The Pilates Method Alliance has a certification program similar to the board certification process used in other areas of health care. Don't hesitate to ask a potential instructor what kind of training and certification he or she has received.

Joseph Pilates invented some novel pieces of equipment for his exercises, and some Pilates studios or health clubs may offer individual or small group classes that utilize these creations. The most common piece of equipment, the *reformer,* is based on Joe's early use of springs and hospital beds for rehabilitation. In some cases classes are done without any equipment at all. These are referred to as *mat classes,* as they are performed on an exercise mat on the floor.

Here are two of Joe's most famous exercises:

- *The Hundred:* Start by lying flat on the floor. Inhale while raising your legs off the floor, keeping them straight with toes pointed. Lift your head and extend your arms several inches over your thighs. Exhale while pulsing your arms up and down for five counts, and then inhale while pulsing for five counts. Keep going until you reach one hundred counts or as far as you can go.

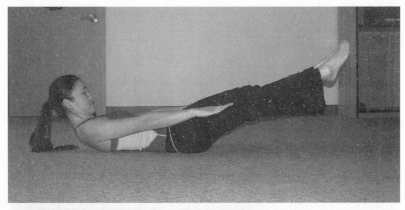

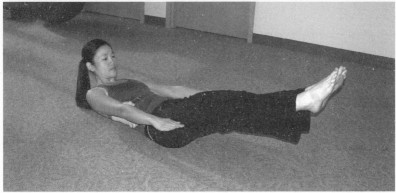

- *The Teaser:* Proper form is essential with this exercise. Start off sitting upright with your legs pointing straight ahead and resting on the floor. Gradually roll down onto your back while lifting your legs and head, with your arms at your side. Inhale as you lift your torso off the ground and raise your arms up in a parallel line with your already raised legs. Exhale while returning to the reclined position while keeping your legs lifted off the ground. Beginners should first try this maneuver under the supervision of a trainer or physical therapist.

Both of these exercises require strong core muscles that should stay engaged the entire time. Without strong core muscles, you will

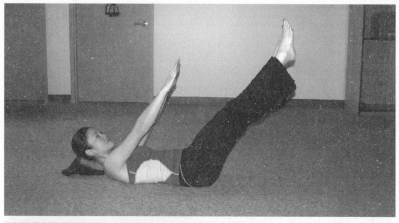

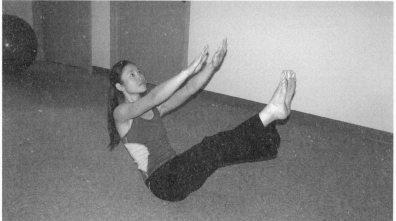

start to use other muscles to hold the body up, like neck and shoulder muscles, which can become overly tense.

Check with Your Doctor!

For chronic pain sufferers, these alternative kinds of exercise can be valuable additions to standard medical treatments. Tai chi or qigong classes are an excellent place to start because they typically involve slow-paced, easy movements. As for yoga, if you're a newcomer, I recommend gentle or restorative classes, which focus on relaxation and easy stretches. No matter what form of exercise you choose, be sure to check with your doctor before beginning any new exercise class or program. If you are suffering from a recent injury or having a painful flare-up, you may need to wait until your body has healed sufficiently before you start something new. When you do begin taking classes, tell the instructor about your injury or condition so that he or she can modify or eliminate certain exercises for you when necessary.

As always, caution is essential. It's also a good idea to start at a beginner's level and take it easy at first, especially if you're starting an entirely new exercise program. See how your body responds, especially in the injured or painful area. If a certain stretch or movement causes pain, stop immediately.

It Never Gets Stale

The explanations and examples in this chapter are just the tip of the iceberg. You can spend years studying, practicing, and gaining ever greater health benefits from Eastern movement therapies, as well as their Western "cousin," Pilates. I have come to appreciate all of them for the endless opportunities for growth and changes they offer. Even though I get a year older every April, I feel that I keep getting *more* flexible thanks to these disciplines. At a time in my life when most guys my age are getting stiffer, I'm actually moving in the opposite direction, and the good feeling that results makes me want to improve my physical, emotional, and spiritual health in other ways as well. I hate to think what the state of my health would be right now without these timeless practices.

Complementary alternative medical treatments, those discussed here as well as others, comprise a valuable part of my core healing strategies. For chronic pain sufferers they fill in the blanks overlooked by some of traditional medical treatments. I urge you to discard your "I'm a patient" mind-set; to think of yourself as being whole, healthy, and at peace with life; and to study Eastern health ideas and practices so that you can avail yourself of the best of Eastern and Western medicine.

CHAPTER 18

Common Western Medical Treatments for Chronic Pain

Modern medicine is nothing short of amazing. Doctors, paramedics, and nurses perform life-saving miracles every day. The pills we prescribe and the scalpels we wield are powerful weapons that can repair torn parts, control "misbeating hearts," and save failing organs. Today people recover from certain types of cancers that were fatal just a few years ago and go on to lead normal lives. Remarkable medical breakthroughs are constantly occurring that can both lengthen life and boost its quality for years to come. This incredible arsenal of technology and knowledge has given us the ability to knock out disease, heal ailing or broken bodies, and diminish suffering.

It's almost as if doctors today have the *Midas touch*. King Midas, of Greek mythology fame, was given the magical power of turning anything he touched into gold. While he was overjoyed at the prospect of creating wealth beyond his wildest dreams, Midas hadn't thought through the implications of his wish. It soon became apparent that turning *everything* he touched into gold was not only impractical, it could be more of a curse than a blessing. Midas inadvertently turned his own son into a golden statue, and every time the wealthy ruler tried to eat, his food turned into gold before he could get it into his mouth. He had to beg to get the spell lifted before his whole world turned into cold, hard metal. Obviously, if Midas had thought about it more carefully, he would have been more specific about which things he wanted to become gold.

Modern Western medicine has a lot in common with King Midas. It can accomplish great things, but if used indiscriminately can wreak havoc. The key, of course, is to know when to bring on the magic and when to leave things alone. Like Midas, physicians must be very careful with what they do. The prescriptions they

225

write, procedures they perform, and words they speak can hurt as much as they help. But you, the patient, also play an important part in deciding when the Midas touch is warranted and when it isn't. You're the one who decides whether or not to accept a medication, surgery, or other treatment. You needn't rely solely on your doctor to make these choices, for you can gather information from your doctor, other health professionals, your spouse, friends, books, magazines, and the Internet to help you make these very important decisions. The challenge, of course, lies in figuring out which treatments to embrace and which to avoid. What makes this especially difficult is that you are a unique individual, so what works best for someone else may not be best for you.

This chapter outlines the treatments you will most likely need to make decisions about at one point or another. The recommendations I give about various medications and medical techniques are based on information provided by well-respected studies and think tanks. It won't tell you what is absolutely right for you, but it's a good place to start.

Medications
Certain types of medications work better with one type of pain, while other types may be more effective with a different type of pain. As noted previously, pain experts divide pain into acute, chronic, and cancer pain. *Chronic* pain can be broken up into different subcategories, including nerve pain (also known as neuropathic pain), musculoskeletal pain (pain involving muscles and bones; examples include fibromyalgia and compression fractures), and arthritis pain. This chapter's review of medications, as well as surgeries and procedures, will focus primarily on these three types of chronic pain.

Neuropathic Pain Medications
Neuropathic pain refers to a major subtype of chronic pain caused by damage to a nerve, or a dysfunction within the nervous system.

The word *neuropathic* means "pathology in the nerves." Nerve pain can be described as burning, sharp, shooting, electrical, or pins and needles, depending on the circumstances and particular type of problem. There are many types of nerve pain syndromes; in fact, whole books are written about neuropathic pain and some of its most typical and vexing syndromes. One particular type often studied is *diabetic neuropathy.* People with diabetes have a tendency to lose small nerve fibers in distant locations like the feet. When this happens, they develop a burning pain in their feet that can spread up the legs.

While research often focuses on the diabetic neuropathy model, keep in mind that the most common causes of nerve pain are related to problems with the spine. This includes the classic example of sciatica, where a nerve gets "pinched" in the lower back, causing pain to shoot down the back of the leg. And also remember that just because a treatment shows good results against one type of neuropathic pain, it is not necessarily a magic weapon for all chronic pain problems.

The major scientific organization dedicated to the study and treatment of pain is the International Association of the Study of Pain (IASP), and our national chapter is known as the American Pain Society (APS). These organizations put together a group of their experts and published updated, evidence-based medicine guidelines on how to treat neuropathic pain. Here is a summary of their neuropathic pain medication recommendations:

1. First Line Medications
Best options for most cases and should be tried first.
- **Tricyclic antidepressants:** These medications increase the levels of certain brain chemicals that regulate pain signals and improve mood.
  - o   amitryptiline (trade name Elavil)
  - o   nortryptiline (Pamelor)
  - o   desipramine (Norpramin)

- **Selective serotonin and norepinephrine reuptake inhibitors:**
  These medications increase levels of the neurotransmitters
  norepinephrine and serotonin in the central nervous system.
    o duloxetine (Cymbalta)
    o venlafaxine (Effexor)
- **Calcium channel ligands:** These medications change the flow
  of positively charged calcium ions, which can quiet irritated
  nerves.
    o gabapentin (Neurontin)
    o pregabalin (Lyrica)
- **Topical lidocaine** (lidocaine patches): This can reduce the
  activation of superficial pain fibers on the skin.

2. Second Line Medications

Used for acute episodes (flare-ups) and for nerve pain associated
with cancer.
- **Opioid-based medications:** Opioids work by attaching to
  specific receptors in the brain, spinal cord, and body, where
  they block the transmission of pain messages to the brain. See
  chapter 4 for a list of opioid-based medications.

3. Third Line Medications

Can be tried for chronic nerve pain when first line options have
not been successful.
- **Antiepileptics:** These medications stabilize the flow of charged
  ions across nerve membranes.
    o topiramate (Topamax)
    o carbamazepine (Tegretol)
    o lamotrigine (Lamictal)
- **Antidepressants:** These medications increase the levels of
  certain brain chemicals that regulate pain signals and improve
  mood.
    o buproprion (Wellbutrin)

- o   citalopram (Celexa)
- o   paroxetine (Paxil)
- **Miscellaneous:** Medications to reduce extra nerve excitation.
  - o   mexiletine (Mexitil)
  - o   topical capsaicin (Capsagel)

The IASP and ASP note that these medications should be part of a comprehensive approach that includes nonpharmacologic treatments. Keep in mind that all drugs have potential side effects that may limit their usefulness.

Fibromyalgia Medications

Fibromyalgia is a syndrome associated with inflammation of the connective tissue (the muscles, tendons, and ligaments), which brings about widespread musculoskeletal tenderness and an elevated sensitivity to pain. Symptoms include chronic pain, stiffness, fatigue, insomnia, and mood changes like depression. Basically, fibromyalgia sufferers feel like they ache all over. No one knows what causes the syndrome, but it's often triggered by stress, other diseases, infections, injury, or a lack of sleep.

Fibromyalgia has received increased attention over the last few years because the FDA has approved two medications to treat its symptoms. When pregabalin (Lyrica), the first of the two, was approved, its manufacturer, Pfizer, launched a lot of advertising and marketing. The second of the two, duloxetine, also known as Cymbalta, was likewise anointed by the FDA. These two medications do not act directly on inflamed muscles, and their mechanisms of action in fibromyalgia are not clear, but they may work by influencing the processing of pain within the pain matrix.

With the exception of pregabalin and duloxetine, the choice of medications to treat fibromyalgia is usually based on the doctor's intuitive response to the patient's physical and emotional complaints, rather than on the results of scientific studies. This is why many fibromyalgia sufferers take a wide array of prescribed drugs. (Beware the King Midas syndrome!)

Osteoarthritis Medications

Osteoarthritis (OA) is a disease that causes the breakdown of cartilage in the joints, leading to friction between bone ends, inflammation, pain, and sometimes bone spurs. Some twenty-seven million adults currently suffer from OA, which is a major contributor to declining function in the elderly. The increase in the number of obese people in our society can only mean that the incidence of OA will continue to rise, for excess weight can put pressure on the knees and other weight-bearing joints and worsen OA.

The symptomatic use of nonsteroidal anti-inflammatory drugs (NSAIDs) to diminish the swelling and discomfort of involved joints is a standard practice. There are numerous medications in this class of drugs, including ibuprofen, naproxen, diclofenac, and salicylate. Pharmaceutical companies are now coming out with topical versions with the hope of improving results and limiting side effects. Patients often ask me which of these medications is best. There really isn't an answer to that question, for results vary from person to person.

Some NSAIDs are sold over the counter, and most doctors freely prescribe the rest, so they are used as commonly as vitamins and toothpaste in many households. They aren't without side effects, though, including nausea, diarrhea, constipation, and fluid retention. More serious side effects include excessive bleeding, ulcers, and liver and kidney failure. It is now estimated that one hundred thousand people are hospitalized annually due to the effects of NSAIDs and approximately sixteen thousand die each year, which equals the number of Americans who die annually from AIDS.

NSAIDS reduce pain and swelling by inhibiting the action of an enzyme known as cyclooxygenase (COX). Inhibiting COX has the effect of slowing down the production of substances that create inflammation. This also interferes with the cascade of events that allows blood to clot, which is why NSAID side effects may include bleeding ulcers. The body has a few different types of COX enzymes. Newer NSAIDS that more specifically block the COX-2 enzymes are called COX-2 inhibitors. These medications are less likely to block the clotting cascade, which makes them a good option for patients who are concerned about bleeding problems like ulcers. The only COX-2 currently available on the market is celecoxib (Celebrex), but more are on the way.

As mentioned earlier, there are many types of arthritis, but osteoarthritis is the most prevalent. Rheumatoid arthritis occurs when the body's own immune system starts to attack its own joints, causing pain and inflammation. Medications specifically designed to halt the body's autoimmune attack against itself are frequently tried to ease the pain associated with rheumatoid arthritis.

Cancer Pain Medications

Cancer pain is usually differentiated as a separate branch of pain medicine, even though some of the recommended treatments can overlap with chronic pain management. There is a general consensus about how to optimize the use of medications for cancer pain. Efforts by groups like the World Health Organization have brought to our attention the worldwide undertreatment of cancer pain, which can be triggered by a variety of different causes, and treatments should be directed accordingly. Depending on the type of cancer pain, all the major medication classifications can be potential options, including the anti-inflammatories, acetaminophen, opioids, and the nerve pain medicines mentioned above.

Even in end-of-life care, people can develop tolerances to their opioid pain medications and suffer increased pain (opioid-induced hyperalgesia). This phenomenon creates special challenges for everyone involved. In more complicated cases, many different types of medications may need to be mixed and matched in order to calm things down. At times like this, throwing the kitchen sink at a problem really is in the person's best interest.

Deciding Whether or Not to Take Pain Medication

When making decisions about whether or not to take pain medications, and which ones to choose, be sure to remember the following suggestions:

- *Avoid being a passive patient.* You don't need to agree to every medication that your doctor suggests. Look into the side effects and drug interactions of a medication before you put it into your mouth. Weigh the benefits against the risks and ask how long it's expected that you'll need to take this medication. Ask about other options, both pharmaceutical and alternative.
- *Don't assume new drugs are safer or better than their predecessors.* A lot of research on new drugs never gets published before the FDA approves them. When these unpublished findings are investigated, their results are almost always unfavorable in some way.
- *Think of your body as a temple.* A temple is a place of sacred activity. Be very selective about what enters it.

Ultimately when making a decision about medications, you need to consider many different factors, including possible reactions with other medications you currently take, potential side effects, what type of pain you have (for example, neuropathic or arthritic), out-of-pocket costs, and how it may help or interfere with your ability to function (which includes doing things like driving a car). Listen to your body. If something doesn't feel right, that should be a warning sign that you need to report it to your doctor right away.

Surgery

Doctors have long resorted to the knife to treat certain painful conditions, but the use of many surgeries for the treatment of chronic pain—as opposed to those for acute injuries like fractures and tears—remains controversial. There are still many questions to be answered, even about more common surgeries such as spine surgery. For example, where does low back surgery fit in for the treatment of *chronic low back pain?* And what does your doctor mean by *"good results"?* Most of the patients I talk to believe that good results should mean the pain disappears and doesn't return. But evidence-based medicine does not offer a resounding endorsement of spine surgery as a cure for *chronic pain.*

Let's review some important studies that may help put things in better perspective.

Herniated Disk Surgery

The results of the Spine Patient Outcomes Research Trial (SPORT), which looked at patients with herniated disks, were published in the *Journal of the American Medical Association* in 2006.[16] The SPORT study involved 501 patients at 13 centers in 11 states. Some of the patients had surgery to repair the disks; others did not. After two years, the researchers found that the results of the surgery were positive overall, but most patients improved during that time whether they had the surgery or not. In other words, there was no proof that surgery was any more effective than simply waiting for the back to heal on its own.

Spinal Stenosis Surgery

In a follow-up SPORT study[17] the focus was on surgery for spinal stenosis, which is a narrowing within the spinal canal that develops over time as spinal structures degenerate. This condition is the most common reason for spine surgery in people over sixty-five. The surgery involves the removal of disk material and/or bone to open up space for the nerve roots. In this study some of the vol-

16   Weinstein, J.N., Tosteson, T.D., Lurie, J.D., et al. "Surgical vs. nonoperative treatment for lumbar disk herniation: The Spine Patient Outcomes Research (SPORT): A randomized trial." *JAMA* 2006; 296:2441–2450.

17   Tosteson, A.N.A., Jurie, J.D., Tosteson, T.D., et al. "Surgical treatment of spinal stenosis with and without degenerative spondylolisthesis: Cost-effectiveness after 2 years." *Ann. Intern. Med.* 2008; 149(12):845–853.

unteers underwent surgery, while others did not. After two years the researchers found that those who had the surgery had a better outcome than those who didn't have it. However, the nonsurgery patients *didn't* worsen during this time; either they improved or they remained the same.

Note: The SPORT studies were *not* specifically chronic pain studies. They involved people who had experienced pain for as little as six to twelve weeks, while chronic pain, by definition, is present for at least six months.

Spinal Fusion Surgery

Spinal fusion surgeries typically involve putting hardware into the spine to stabilize it. Compared to surgeries for herniated disks or spinal stenosis, spinal fusion surgery is much more invasive, costly, and requires a much longer recovery time

While spinal fusion surgery may be useful for lower back trauma, spinal deformities where the spine has abnormal curves, or when the back is not stable, it has not been shown to be any more effective in reducing low back pain than aggressive rehabilitation plus time. The evidence does not support the use of spinal fusion solely for the treatment of chronic low back pain, although it is commonly used for this purpose. Also troubling is the fact that spinal fusions often need to be repeated; perhaps as many as one in five is repeated within a couple of years of the first surgery.

Hip and Knee Replacement

It might be more accurate to refer to joint replacement surgery as joint *rebuilding* surgery. The surgeon tries to maintain the integrity of the natural joint and rebuild it by cutting away diseased tissue, resurfacing certain areas, or replacing a part of the joint—say the socket of a ball-and-socket joint. Or, in some cases, the entire joint is replaced with artificial parts. The results can be terrific: Joint replacements typically relieve pain, improve joint stability, and recover mobility, which can help restore a person's independence and general outlook on life. However, joint replacements are not without complications, which can include blood clots, nerve damage in the area surrounding the joint, and legs that are uneven in length. Joints can wear out, as well. Hips typically last ten to fifteen years and knees about twenty years. Then the surgery must be repeated.

Surgery for Trigeminal Neuralgia
Trigeminal neuralgia involves severe shooting or jabbing pain on one side of the face in the areas served by the trigeminal nerve, such as the jaw, cheek, gums, lips, and teeth. It's most commonly seen in women over fifty and is typically caused by a blood vessel that exerts pressure on the trigeminal nerve inside the skull. When the standard nerve pain medications are not effective, surgery may be an option. While there are different techniques, the most common approach is to enter the skull just behind the ear, find the problem, and decompress it.

Most studies show favorable results with this surgery, but it is a delicate procedure with all the risks that can be expected when operating around important nerves and blood supply to the brain.

Surgery for Chronic Pelvic Pain
Another problem that primarily affects women is *chronic pelvic pain.* There are many causes of this pain, but most cases are poorly understood and difficult to treat. Treatment may include pain-relieving medications, hormone treatments, antidepressants, trigger point injections, counseling, and, in some cases, surgery. The surgeries may include the removal of pelvic adhesions or endometriosis deposits or, in more severe cases, a full hysterectomy. Yet in 2005 the Cochrane Review found no evidence to support surgical treatments in the case of chronic pelvic pain. They found that both a multidisciplinary approach and progesterone therapy were more effective.

Before Agreeing to Any Surgery, Remember . . .

There are so many different factors involved in most chronic pain syndromes, so it is often unrealistic to expect to solve everything with an isolated surgical treatment. With any surgery, it always helps to develop realistic expectations and become well-informed about the recovery process. Ask your doctor to direct you to books and online resources so you can become educated and prepared. It doesn't hurt to ask your surgeon if you can speak with any of his/her patients who have had the same surgery; they can explain what the experience is like from the patient's perspective.

Injections

The use of injections designed to relieve pain has increased substantially over the last two decades, with the sheer number of procedures performed growing as pain management has developed into its own medical specialty. The most common are cortisone-type injections done around the neck or low back. Research shows that these procedures can be effective in reducing pain symptoms, but the results wear off over time if the problem doesn't eventually get better on its own.

For pain radiating down an arm or leg due to a bulging disk, your physician may consider an epidural injection. If the problem is new or subacute (less than six months duration), an epidural cortisone injection can reduce discomfort during the natural healing process.

If the problem is chronic, however, the injection can still provide relief, but there is a good chance the effects will wear off over time and the pain will return. In some cases, such as with an elderly patient with spinal stenosis who can't tolerate surgery or other treatments, periodic epidural injections might be a reasonable option.

Some of the other procedures commonly performed for pain relief generally show similar results. They may provide short-term symptomatic relief for chronic problems that flare up, but they do not "cure" the old condition. They can also relieve the symptoms of acute injuries that are likely to heal over time and with appropriately chosen interventions, such as a shoulder joint inflamed from bursitis.

There is not an abundance of scientific evidence to back the use of cortisone injections, so they are often performed because we *think* they might help or have worked well for other patients with similar issues.

Over the last several years, procedures called vertebroplasty and kyphoplasty have been proven to relieve pain and strengthen spinal vertebrae that have suffered compression fractures (breaks that occur within the round body of the vertebra). However, some recently published studies have questioned their effectiveness. The major cause of compression fractures in the back is osteoporosis. The National Osteoporosis Foundation estimates that ten million Americans have osteoporosis, resulting in seven hundred thousand compression fractures to the spinal column each year, at an annual cost of fourteen billion dollars. Not only do compression fractures cause excruciating pain, they can lead to significant functional impairments like reduced mobility and difficulty breathing. For both vertebroplasty and kyphoplasty, a cement material is injected into the area of the injury, stabilizing the back and usually eliminating a lot of the discomfort.

Although both of these procedures can be helpful, they are not without risk. The cement material can leak from the vertebra as it is being injected, possibly causing nerve damage or a pulmonary embolism, a blood clot that can move into the lungs and threaten your life. These are not common complications, but they do happen. These procedures can also cause new fractures to occur. For these reasons, vertebroplasty and kyphoplasty should be performed by experienced physicians and only if you have quick access to a major medical center where these potential side effects can be treated.

Interventions and Medications Aren't the Whole Answer

This brief review is designed to give you a basic idea of the medications, surgeries, and injections typically used for common chronic pain syndromes. This does not suggest that I am predicting the outcome of your own unique situation. I'm simply passing on evidence-based information to help you put things in perspective.

Chronic pain impacts everything imaginable, from personal relationships to physical activities and career success. Even opioids, the strongest painkillers in existence, don't necessarily control chronic pain over time. Effective treatment must go beyond focusing on just making a diagnosis and applying the "cure." Instead it must take into consideration the needs of the whole person. When the exact causes of the pain are not entirely clear, doctors may be tempted to work backward by starting with the treatment options, like injections, and developing a plan based on what is available rather than doing the hard work of understanding the needs of the patient. This is no surprise, for *when you have a hammer, everything can look like a nail.*

You are likely surrounded by accomplished doctors and health care providers who hold the keys to powerful treatments, like strong medications and innovative surgeries that can reconstruct parts of the body. These treatments can be very tempting. Remember, however, that you are more than a pain generator or a disease. You may need to take the initiative and explore different options, like modern psychology and physical rehabilitation; join a needed charity; take tai chi at your community center; or get a group together to see a new show or exhibit. All of these therapies and activities can play a valuable role in healing the different faces of what hurts.

For many of us the best results come when we combine the right amounts of traditional and alternative treatments. That seems to be true in the case of Trent, whose left foot was crushed by a heavy truck in a bizarre work-related injury. The accident fractured a bone in his foot and caused nerve damage. Surgery was required so the bones could heal properly and give the foot a better chance to function correctly. Unfortunately, while the surgeon successfully repaired the broken bone and cleaned up the scar tissue, Trent's burning nerve pain persisted without improvement. He had to give up exercising and sports. Even walking was painful—not only because of the original pain, but because of new pains and stiffness caused by the exaggerated limp he used to reduce his foot pain. One of his doctors tried putting him on the medication gabapentin, which seemed to eliminate some of the burning pain caused by the nerve damage.

Although Trent benefitted from the surgeries, medications, and special nerve blocks he received, bearing weight on his left foot remained very difficult because of the pain it caused. He made some progress, but not enough to stay on his feet long enough to go to work or walk across a shopping mall. At that point if his doctors had thrown more medications and surgeries at him, I don't think it would have really helped. Fortunately his doctors suggested he talk to me about possible alternative treatments. As he learned about things like breathing, flare-up management, and pacing activities, and worked on improving his gait and body mechanics, Trent was gradually able to manage the pain in his foot well enough so that he could stand upright long enough to start exercising and working again. All the treatments he received played a valuable role in his progress.

Understanding what modern medicine can and can't do to help you with your pain helps you take advantage of breakthrough therapies, avoid treatments that you don't need, and focus some of your valuable time on useful alternative healing strategies. And there's one more thing you can do: sleep well. Getting the proper amount of sleep at night is associated with a longer life expectancy. The next chapter is dedicated solely to this area of great frustration for those with chronic pain.

CHAPTER 19

Lights Out: Simple Ways to Better Sleep

Sleep problems are the second most common complaint (after pain) that I hear from my patients. That's no surprise, for we treasure those hours of sleep. From the moment we enter the world, sleep is a source of comfort and relief from the trials and tribulations of wet, smelly diapers and suction bulbs shoved up our noses. As infants, sleeping in our mothers' arms was pure bliss. As we get older, sleep offers both a respite from the world and the promise of rejuvenation.

It seems unfair, then, that the more pain we have and the longer it lasts, the harder it becomes to get a good night's sleep. Insomnia seems to follow pain like a tail on a cat. I don't know which upsets my patients more: the feeling of fatigue or the denial of their unalienable right to a good night's sleep.

Of course sleep problems are not unusual; if anything they are quite common, even among those who don't have pain. The National Sleep Foundation estimates that about seventy million Americans currently experience sleep problems and forty million have chronic sleep disorders. We pay a hefty price in aggravation, fatigue, and cold hard cash for our sleep problems. According to the Sleep Research Project at the University of Alabama, we spend a cool one billion dollars every year on prescription and over-the-counter sleep medications.

We spend so much because sleep is important. Adequate sleep— but not too much—is necessary for good health. While seven to eight hours of sleep per night is associated with longer life, those who get fewer than seven hours, or more than eight and a half hours, tend to be less healthy and live shorter lives. With inadequate sleep, stress hormones such as cortisol increase, triggering inflammation. This impairs the immune system, making us more susceptible to colds and flu.

Both motor and mental acuity suffer when we are sleep deprived, which can lead to dangerous human errors and accidents. Studies done on test subjects with occupations associated with sleep deprivation—including pilots, truck drivers, and medical residents—typically show a greater risk for fatigue-related mistakes and crashes. Accidents related to sleepiness result in lost lives and billions of dollars in costs. Psychomotor impairment due to sleep deprivation, as seen on tests like driving performance, can resemble that seen with blood alcohol levels between .05 and .1 percent.[18]

Sleep, on the other hand, helps to restore both mind and body. The body's engines are able to slow down and cool off when we sleep, decreasing the metabolic processes, heart rate, respiration, digestion, and body temperature. Sleep can also be a time of increased healing from injuries or, in children, a time of accelerated growth.

Why Is Sleep So Elusive?

We often hear that sleep requirements vary from person to person, and while I'm sure there is some variability due to genetics, I recommend seven to eight hours per night. Unfortunately, it seems that we in the twenty-first century sleep less, on average, than our forefathers did. There are a number of reasons for this, including the fact that sleep cycles shorten in old age. If you sleep eight hours a night when you're in your thirties, there's a good chance you'll be sleeping seven hours or less by the time you reach seventy-five. And since folks live longer now than they did one hundred years ago, the average amount of sleep we Americans get has decreased.

---

18 Fairclough, S.H., and R. Graham, (1999), "Impairment of Driving Performance Caused by Sleep Deprivation or Alcohol: A Comparative Study." *The Journal of Human Factors and Ergonomics Society,* 41:118–128.

Dawson, D. and K. Reid. "Fatigue, Alcohol and Performance Impairment." *Nature* 1997; 338:235.

Williamson, A.M., and A.M. Feyer. "Moderate Sleep Deprivation Produces Impairments in Cognitive and Motor Performance Equivalent to Legally Prescribed Levels of Alcohol Intoxication." *Occupational and Environmental Medicine,* 2000; 57:649–655.

The invention of electricity has had a big impact on our sleeping habits, too. Before people had electric lights, they typically went to bed once it got dark outside. But now we can light up our homes and cities all night, which makes it possible for us to stay up hours longer than our ancestors did. And during this time we're often engaged in stimulating activities like watching television, talking on the phone, sending and receiving text messages, listening to music, playing computer games, surfing the Internet, and reading e-mail. All of this sensory overload makes it harder to achieve a peaceful and lasting sleep. On top of this, our modern culture deemphasizes the value of sleep, as evidenced by the surge in popularity of caffein-ated energy drinks like Red Bull. Designed to create a jolt of activ-ity, these drinks are often consumed by young adults and teenagers wishing to stay up late cramming for tests or partying. Energy drinks generate over two billion dollars in annual sales, so somebody out there just doesn't want us to get cozy in our pajamas.

Then there are those who want to cram too many activities into each day, so they sacrifice sleep to get more done. These are the high-octane overachievers who rush quickly from one activity to another and work long hours. They believe that cutting out an hour or two of sleep at night will help them get more work done, so they drink coffee all day to help keep them going.

All of these can change or disrupt our *circadian rhythms,* the innate twenty-four-hour clock that dictates the ebb and flow of bio-logical processes like hunger and sleep. External factors like bright lights, noise, and caffeine modify the circadian rhythms, which mean they affect when you want to eat dinner or wake up in the morning. Exposing living creatures to increased periods of light can lead to shorter sleep cycles, just as exposure to darkness leads to longer sleep cycles.

Visualize a casino. Inside there are no windows, so you are not exposed to natural sunlight or darkness. Lights and bells flash con-stantly, providing continuous stimulation to the eyes and ears. The floor plan keeps you wandering from one gaming area to another, and exits are not always easy to find. There are no day and night cycles inside casinos—just a state of constant stimulation designed to override your circadian rhythms and keep you gambling without interruption. If you have this type of atmosphere in your bedroom or home, you may not want to sleep as much as you should. If your TV, computer, text messages, cell phone, iPod, video game console, and other devices are constantly beckoning you, you've unwittingly created an environment filled with casino-like stimulation that makes it tempting to cut back on your sleep.

Chronic pain can also be a huge obstacle to enjoying quality sleep. Moving a painful body part can trigger a pain reaction that automatically wakes you up. Yet trying to lie still in bed can cause stiffness and more pain. The mood changes associated with pain, like depression and anxiety, can also bring on insomnia. Clearly, pain is the enemy of sleep. Luckily you can do much to set the stage for a good night's sleep.

Beyond Counting Sheep: Nine Tips to Better Sleep

Often the next sentence I hear from patients after they tell me they sleep poorly is, "What can you give me to help me sleep?" While they are asking me this, they might be holding a super-size double-trouble latte that they absolutely *needed* before their appointment. In other words they're saying, "Doc, I need something to put me to sleep at night and something else to wake me up in the morning."

A large percentage of patients with chronic pain take regular medications to help them sleep, and it's easy to understand why. Patients expect their doctors to do something about their insomnia and fatigue, and doctors feel pressured to respond to their needs. The likely outcome is that patients will leave the doctor's office with a prescription for something to help them sleep. However, research on the treatment of sleep disorders consistently shows that improved sleep hygiene, not sleeping pills, is the most effective way to improve sleep.

Helping patients improve their sleep hygiene means teaching them about the things that facilitate or hinder sleep. Unfortunately, this type of training can't be squeezed into a brief office visit, nor is it something most physicians are accustomed to doing. Instead they prescribe sleeping pills. But not only are these pills likely less effective, they can have significant side effects, too, like causing Grandma, who took something to help her sleep, to wander around the neighborhood in the middle of the night wondering where she is.

I believe the key to improving sleep revolves around what we know about circadian rhythms. If you can make changes in your environment and lifestyle that allow this natural process to take over, then you stand a better chance of getting the sleep you need. Remember: Circadian rhythms depend on exposure to daylight and darkness in a predictable pattern. Fluctuations in your habits can prevent you from getting into a rhythm, which throws off your sleep schedule. In other words, don't let your brain feel like it is in a casino.

Here are some tips for improving your sleep hygiene:

1. **Create a calming environment in your bedroom.** Try to make your sleeping environment as sleep friendly as possible by blocking out noise with a fan or white noise machine, darkening the room with blackout shades or heavy drapes, making sure that your mattress and pillow are comfortable, and that the room is cool but not too cold.

2. **Exercise regularly.** Exercise is a great stress reliever, and studies have shown that those who exercise regularly sleep longer and more deeply than those who don't. But don't exercise too late in the day, and certainly not right before you crawl into bed! This can cause a surge in energy-producing hormones like adrenaline and raise your body temperature, which must drop to a certain level before you can fall asleep and stay asleep.

3. **Avoid caffeinated beverages after noon.** Caffeine is a stimulant, and the highs and lows created by caffeinated drinks

can rev you up enough to keep you awake. If you seem to be caffeine sensitive, stay away from beverages like coffee, black tea, soda, chocolate, and cocoa, as well as medications that contain caffeine (particularly headache remedies), after noon. Consider substituting noncaffeinated beverages such as decaf coffee or tea, herbal teas, or plain water and using medications that don't contain caffeine.

4. **Don't eat heavy meals late at night.** Your body expends a lot of energy digesting food, especially proteins and fats. When you have a meal or a large snack too close to bedtime, you increase both bodily activity and temperature, confusing your body as to whether it should be falling asleep or waking up. Eat your evening meal a good two to three hours before bedtime and limit liquids in the evening to cut back on those middle-of-the-night trips to the bathroom that disrupt your sleep.

5. **Spend time outdoors during the day.** You need exposure to light to create and maintain circadian rhythms. Not only does a lack of exposure to daylight throw off your sleep cycles, it can be downright depressing. That's because when you're exposed to bright light, your brain starts making a neurotransmitter called serotonin, which wakes you up and makes you feel alert, energetic, and happy. Serotonin, in turn, is the raw material for another neurotransmitter called melatonin, which shifts your body into lower gear, making you feel drowsy and getting you ready for sleep. Without enough serotonin, it's hard to make sufficient melatonin when it's time to fall asleep.

6. **Avoid alcohol before bedtime.** While it may seem that the sedating effects of alcohol will help you slow down and fall asleep faster, alcohol actually contributes to poor quality sleep. Drinking alcohol before bedtime will disrupt your normal sleep cycles and keep you from getting the restorative kind of sleep you need. As a result you'll feel tired, dull, and possibly hungover in the morning.

7. **Wind down about an hour before bedtime.** Some people race around, doing chores and preparing for the next day right up until they fall into bed exhausted. Then they're surprised (and annoyed) when they can't fall asleep! But the body needs some time to make the transition from being awake to being asleep. Take the time to wind down at the end of the day; start easing in to the mood about an hour before it's time to sleep. Turn off the television, computers, and cell phone. Dim the lights (or at least avoid bright lights), take a nice long bath, engage in quiet conversation, do progressive relaxation exercises, make love, or do anything else that can help you relax and get ready for sleep.

8. **Go to bed and wake up at regularly scheduled times.** Although you may love the idea of sleeping in on the weekends, this can disrupt your internal clock and throw off your sleep schedule. So choose the times that work best for your needs, remembering that the goal is to get seven to eight hours of sleep every night, and try to get up and go to bed at the same times every day. This will create an internal rhythm that increases your chances of sleeping well.

9. **Use your bed for sleep or sex only.** It's tempting to use your bed for all kinds of activities, including watching TV, paying bills, talking on the phone, reading, and playing with the kids. But the more things you do in bed, the more your bed will be associated with activity. You want your bed to be associated with relaxation, so only use it for making love and sleeping. Then, when you come to bed, your mind will automatically realize it's time to relax.

Falling Asleep Again

We've all lived through this scenario: You fall asleep with no problem, only to wake up in the middle of the night and have trouble dropping off to sleep again. You lie there waiting for sleep and end up thinking about aches and pains, work, relationship problems, how to decorate the living room, and on and on. Two hours later, you may still be lying there waiting for sleep.

When this happens, try doing some simple breathing exercises to quiet the mind. Lie on your back and focus only on the motion of the breath as it makes the chest and belly rise and fall. Inhale slowly and deeply; then slowly exhale. Sometimes I hold my inhalation for five counts with each cycle. When I do these exercises, I often find that I fall asleep again within a few minutes.

If you find that you are still wide awake after lying in bed for half an hour, get up and take a break from the whole sleep process. Go into another room and engage in a calming (even boring) activity like reading something dull or folding laundry. Then, when you feel like you might be able to fall asleep again, go back to bed. The idea is to keep from associating your bed with sleeplessness. If you lie awake in bed for more than a half hour on too many consecutive nights, you can develop anxieties about sleeplessness and may dread going to bed. So don't lie there for too long!

Even if you have perfect sleep hygiene and do everything right, there may still be nights when you just can't sleep well. That's when you need to stay calm and keep things in perspective. Sleeplessness can rapidly produce feelings of anxiety, and then panic over not sleeping sets in. Once this occurs it is much harder for you to reach a relaxed state where you can nod off to sleep again. This anxiety can spill over to the next night and the night after that, which means it becomes harder and harder to find restful sleep. As is the case with most things, worrying is counterproductive. Try to remain calm and patient with your sleep hygiene strategies and you'll probably find that good sleep is not the elusive goal you thought it was!

Sweet dreams . . .

CHAPTER 20

At Home: Helping Your Family Help You

I suspect most people have spilled something hot on themselves, like a cup of coffee, at one time or another. I know I have. Let's say you have a cup of Starbuck's finest in your hands, and you accidentally spill it in your lap. How you react to that heated mishap has a lot to do with where it happens. In other words, the action you take after you spill the cup of coffee can be quite different depending on the situation. Here are several scenarios to consider:

1. You are still inside the coffee shop when the cup slips and you spill it down your leg. It feels painfully hot, but there are a lot of people in line. Feeling embarrassed, you try to downplay it in hopes that no one will notice. You grab a napkin and go outside to a private spot to wipe off your skirt or slacks.
2. Somebody bumps into you and the coffee spills on you while you are still in the coffee shop. You get angry at that person and express your displeasure verbally. This time everybody notices.
3. You are all alone in your car when you spill the coffee on your leg. You let out a four-letter expletive directed toward yourself for letting that happen.
4. While at work you accidentally spill the coffee all over your desk and yourself. You are most concerned with protecting the papers on your desk and worry about your own discomfort only after you have saved whatever you can on your desk.

In all five of these scenarios, the coffee is equally hot and the burn should be equally painful, yet the reactions are all distinctly different. But each response is unique only because of the environment in which it took place. This little example shows how physical location, the presence of people, and the specific situation directly impact how we feel about what happens to us and how we react.

Most of us are heavily influenced by our home environment—our spouses, partners, children, parents, cats, dogs, plants, and anything else that is alive and takes up space in our homes. Our opinions, philosophies, activities, and religious preferences are all heavily impacted by the people we live and spend time with. They can have a powerful impact on our ability to heal and grow—and handle chronic pain.

Two Sides of the Same Coin

Scientists have debated the importance of genes versus environment, or *nature versus nurture,* for many years.

Each of us has a unique genetic code. Not only do your chromosomes determine the color of your eyes, the shape of your nose, and the feistiness or gentleness of your personality, they also play a role in determining what types of diseases you may get. The messages carried in your genes are known as *traits*. For example, you can't have blue eyes without a trait for blue eyes somewhere in your genetic makeup.

The *expression* of certain traits, however, is influenced by the environment in which you exist. Our country is experiencing an epidemic of type 2 diabetes, which occurs when the body becomes resistant to its own insulin. This form of diabetes has a basis in genetics: You must have the "diabetes potential" in your genes in order to develop the disease. However, even though our genes haven't changed in the past several generations, a much higher percentage of the population is now getting this disease because of the obesity-enhancing milieu in which they exist. This milieu includes physical inactivity, high-glycemic diets, and an overabundance of calories.

We can see the nature versus nurture drama play out among the Pima Indians, who live in an area that straddles the United States and Mexico. The Pima Indians living in Arizona have the highest rate of diabetes in the world (50 percent!), while their cousins in Mexico, who share the same genes, have a much lower incidence. What's the difference? The most likely culprits are the differences in diet and activity. The Pima in Arizona consume a calorie-rich, high-fat American diet and "enjoy" a relatively sedentary lifestyle, while the Pima in Mexico eat a more traditional diet and are more active. From a genetic point of view both groups are equally susceptible to diabetes, but only one has the high-risk lifestyle for diabetes and the 50 percent rate of type 2 diabetes.

Nature, through genetics, is a very important component of physical ailments, including chronic pain. But nurture, which includes the environment, family, friends, and lifestyle habits, is also very important. *Both* must be addressed when dealing with chronic pain.

Who Are You, Who Are They?

One of the most important things to remember is that you're not the only one who hurts. Undoubtedly your chronic pain has had a tremendous impact on your family. There may be less money coming into the household, and probably more going out to pay for your treatment. Your role in the family may have shifted as you've gone from full-time parent to full-time patient. Everyone else's duties may have doubled as they shoulder some of your old responsibilities and become part-time caregivers. They may resent the attention you're getting or, conversely, be angry if they feel you're foolishly ignoring your pain and encouraging them to do the same. They may be frightened, angry, depressed, resentful, or just plain tired of it all. They may feel guilty because they can't fix your pain, or eager to get the heck out of there and leave it all behind.

Everyone in your family is affected by your chronic pain, and they often take on certain roles in response. They may become *enablers* or *ignorers,* for example, in a subconscious attempt to deal with the difficult situation. You, too, may have taken on a role, perhaps becoming a *hero* or *entitled.* This "cast of characters" in the home environment, including you, can do much to help or hinder your healing. Let's look at some of these characters and see how they influence your overall health and well-being.

The Enabler

Some spouses or partners are, by their nature, very nurturing. When they see that somebody they care about is hurting or injured, they want to do their utmost to help. In no time at all the helpful, loving spouse becomes accustomed to the role of caregiver, assuming a disproportionate amount of responsibility for certain tasks, perhaps taking on all the cleaning and cooking or child care. Problems can creep in when the loving nature of the caregiver starts to interfere with your attempts to resume tasks that you can handle, thereby encouraging you to sink further into inactivity and dependency. In some cases the caregiver may feel it would be cruel to ask you to take on more activities. This over-helpful attitude, which is known as *enabling,* can be physically and emotionally damaging—very damaging.

My team worked with a woman a few years back who had completely stopped using both arms. Not only did her husband do all of the chores around the house, he also handled her self-care activities like combing her hair and wiping her after she went to the bathroom. When we tried to help her regain the use of her hands, he intervened at first and tried to make us stop. He eventually came to realize that it was in his wife's best interest to learn how to care for herself.

Some spouses/partners go beyond enabling and become overbearing, going to all the doctors' appointments, insisting that each doctor finds a cure, doing all the talking, answering all the questions during the history; they can be very controlling. In some cases they'll be the ones to dole out the medicines, giving it when the patient is supposed to have it or when they think the patient needs it.

Spouses/partners aren't the only ones who can become enablers, of course. Any family member or friend can become overly helpful to the point of interfering with the patient's need to do as much as possible for him- or herself as part of the recovery process. And the enabler doesn't have to perform all these "services" in person. For example, a loving adult child might pay for unnecessary round-the-clock care for a parent in pain, buy a very fancy but unnecessary wheelchair, and set up and pay for visits with every pain specialist in town. This may simply enable the chronic pain patient to sink further into passivity and continuing pain.

When a person has an acute injury, such as a broken leg, and cannot do certain things such as bathing, the spouse helps. As the injury heals and is no longer acute, the helping spouse has to make sure he or she avoids becoming an enabler. If he or she continues to do things after the injury heals, it becomes enabling.

The One Who Doesn't Know What to Do

At the opposite end of the spectrum, you'll find the one who doesn't know what to do, the family member or friend who seems to have very little interest in the patient's suffering and is rarely available to help out. These people don't want to hear the patient talk about pain or pills, doctors or exercises. They'll offer little more than a few bland encouragements to stick with your rehabilitation program. They might be turning a deaf ear because they're afraid of facing their own deep-rooted feelings that haven't been processed yet; afraid that their own internal traumas or stressors may come out if they talk about the patient's pain.

The *ignorers* may not be comfortable facing emotional disturbances surrounding chronic pain, like depression, irritability, grief, and anxiety. As a result, they avoid trying to "get too involved" and come across as detached. In other cases they may feel "burned out after hearing the same complaints over and over again." I remember the case of a devoted spouse of one of my long-time patients who eventually broke down psychologically, stopped going to his wife's medical appointments, and began seeing a psychiatrist of his own.

Whatever the reason for the withdrawal, the person with the pain feels even more isolated and hopeless.

The Hero

I see a lot of folks with chronic pain who hide what they're going through and continue with as many of their regular duties and activities as possible. These "push-through-the-pain heroes" are often parents who want to do as much as possible for their children. They have a tendency to overdo activities, overextend themselves, and spend too little time taking care of their own health. Their intentions are great, but their actions drain their energy, ultimately leaving them less able to care for their families than if they were more forthcoming about their needs.

The macho man who focuses on providing for his family and doesn't take care of himself is one such hero. Women are often heroes; the modern woman is expected to have kids, hold down a career, help with homework, feed everyone, and be the glue in the family. In the midst of all of this busy-ness, she is often left without enough time to focus on what *she* needs to get and stay well. There is no balance in the family—or in her life.

Such heroes avoid dealing with stress or their emotions because they are trying to be strong for others. As we have seen before, these hidden feelings eventually "speak" to us through parts of our body, causing more pain in the back, shoulders, and arms, for example. Heroes often try to fight through the pain until they reach their breaking point. The next thing they know, so much tension has built up, perhaps in their hands and arms, that they can barely move the painful parts because they hurt so badly.

Heroes can usually be identified as those who lack balance in their lives. They put a disproportionate amount of their energy into their careers and the lives of their loved ones. They avoid looking after their own needs and health until they start to feel really rotten.

The Entitled Person

Sometimes people with pain feel entitled to be taken care of, especially if they have worked hard for a long time or taken care of others. They believe they deserve to be coddled a bit because of the sacrifices they have made. These entitled people are the flip side of enablers, draining their family and friends dry with requests, pleas, and demands for ever more help.

Recently I treated a woman who had done everything for her family for many years, including holding down a job. She developed chronic pain following a car accident and could not continue being "supermom." She shut down and stopped doing things for everyone else. Her loving family felt that since "Mom did everything for us all these years, we'll take care of her completely, do everything for her." They started to baby her. When she came to us for treatment, she resisted getting better. We later figured out that she subconsciously felt entitled to this special treatment, and if she got better, then she might lose out on it. She wasn't ready to give up the role of the sick person being waited on hand and foot.

Communication, Communication, Communication!

Enabler, ignorer, hero, and entitled: These are among the more common roles I've seen patients, their families, and friends adopt as they grapple with the physical, financial, emotional, social, professional, and other changes brought about by chronic pain. Although these roles may initially seem to be reasonable responses to a difficult situation, in the long run they are harmful. Enabling encourages the chronic pain patient to become weaker, ignoring can trigger resentment and further injury, being a hero can be physically and emotionally damaging and traumatizing to the family when the hero finally collapses, and feeling entitled leads to anger and resentment and eventually strains relationships.

How should you deal with the roles people adopt? By communicating. Communication is key to creating a home environment that will support you as you work to take charge of your pain and maintain control of your life. Communication will help you recognize when someone is taking on a role and help you understand the reasons why.

Always remember that positive changes cannot happen if you hold things inside. In fact, holding things in guarantees problems, because even if you silence your tongue, you're constantly sending out messages in conscious and unconscious ways. Here are examples of what you might do and the resulting messages you send:

- *Isolating yourself:* Simply avoiding others sends a message that can easily be misinterpreted as meaning that you're angry with them.
- *Limping:* The way your body moves tells others how you feel.
- *Grimacing:* You don't see the expressions on your own face unless you happen to look in a mirror, but everyone around you does. Your grimaces can contribute to a negative feeling in the atmosphere.
- *Being irritable*: This can be expressed not only by *what* you say but the *way* you say it. Pay attention to your tone when you communicate.
- *Complaining*: There's a tendency for chronic pain patients to fall into complaining without realizing it. It can be a challenge to explain what is going on objectively, without creating too much negative energy around you.
- *Acting in certain ways:* Family members, especially children, often respond more to what you *do* than what you *say*.

Because a great deal of this communication is unconscious, odds are it will be misunderstood. And misunderstood communication usually leads to more chaos, trouble, and resentment. Holding things in eventually leads to emotional outbursts, which is a less-than-ideal way of communicating with your spouse, partner, children, or other family members.

The best way to communicate about your pain and how it impacts you is to talk it through with the people close to you. Be sure to educate, be positive, keep it light, and listen.

- *Educate:* Provide objective information about your pain so others can get up to speed. Tell them what "went wrong" in your body and how you and your doctor(s) plan to handle it. Don't go into great detail; just give an overview.

- *Emphasize the positive*: Talk about some of the positive things you are doing to manage the problem. Family members usually get really excited when they see positive changes taking place, and that will create even more opportunities to open up new lines of communication.
- *Keep it light:* Talking about ongoing pain can be heavy. Try to balance this with lightness afterward. Perhaps you could all take a walk or go to a funny movie.
- *Listen*: Communication is a two-way street. Be sure to ask them for their views. Listen carefully to what they say, including their biases, and look for ways to clear up misunderstandings.

Talk, and Then . . .

We work hard to create a culture of good health and wellness at our center to nurture patients' progress, but I have seen over and over again how their growth can be stunted when they go home at the end of each day to a negative environment. So now we offer special classes just for family members and spouses to help bridge the gap. Greg Garavanian, a clinical psychologist at our center who oversees this educational program, offers these tips for creating positive change at home:

- Set aside time for direct dialogue. It doesn't have to be a formal discussion with an agenda and gavel; a simple chat will do.
- Avoid whining. Talk instead about helpful things you and others can do.
- Educate family members. Tell them about what you are learning.
- Maintain balance. Pace your activities and try not to overdo things just to make others happy while making yourself miserable.
- Delegate chores appropriately. You don't have to do everything by yourself, and you don't have to do all that you used to do.

Just do as much as you reasonably can, then ask for help from others.

- Engage in regular recreation. If you can no longer participate in your former recreational activities, come up with some new ones that can involve both you and your family.
- Share positive experiences with your spouse or partner. Let him or her know how much fun you're having strolling through the neighborhood, for example, or going to yoga class. Not only does this give your spouse or partner a chance to be supportive, but he or she may join you, which will help improve his or her health and create a bond between the two of you.

Change Is for Everyone

Once you start to change—that is, when your mood has improved, your body has become stronger, or both—your spouse and others close to you will change, too. At first they may seem resistant to a happier and more active you. They will need time to adjust to the fact that you no longer require them to drive you places, shop for you, push you around in a wheelchair, take you to the doctor, and so on, because you can do these things for yourself or they may no longer need to be done at all.

You might think things will simply return to normal, or nearly normal, as you get better, but oddly enough you'll have to talk your way through this phase as well. The fact that you are getting better is yet another change, and all changes bring up the possibility of confusion, anger, fear, and other negative feelings. Perhaps your family won't want you to drive because they are concerned for your safety, or deep down they feel less important because you no longer need them. You may find yourself suddenly wanting to make bold changes in your life, but your family may not yet be ready to move as quickly. Even when the change is something everyone has been hoping for, it can be uncomfortable. The more you communicate, the better you educate them and let them know what you are feeling and the easier it will be for them to come around.

One of my favorite success stories involves a beautiful retired dancer who was suffering from a very painful foot injury. Her husband traveled frequently on business, and she was responsible for looking after her small children. She lived far from our clinic, so it was difficult to convince her to spend a few hours a week there for treatment. As she strove to be a great mom despite the pain, the stress mounted and she eventually agreed to find babysitting help so she could devote some time to her own health. She was also able to educate her husband about her problem so he could better understand her limits and how to help. Once she made these changes at home, she quickly got better. Today she is still a loving, caring mom, but she is free of the old stress and suffers from much less pain.

Despite the challenges that may lie ahead, it is important to remember that it benefits everyone involved when you create an environment at home or at work that supports a healthy lifestyle. At the end of the day this becomes a win-win proposition, which is always the key to any negotiation. Next we will look at aging more closely, and how following a truly healthy lifestyle can help create a "painless retirement."

CHAPTER 21
Aging Gracefully

The anti-aging industry is a large and growing segment of our economy. But the majority of the treatments offered, from skin creams to plastic surgery, are designed simply to make you look younger. Although some anti-aging treatments also stress the importance of what goes into the body, the promised results—characterized by words like *rejuvenate, lift,* and *revitalize*—are mostly cosmetic. While I hope that you'll continue to look great at any age, my real wish is to help you find a path that leads you to feeling wonderful, too. And in order to do that, you'll need to start investing in your health right now. You can't expect to feel like a million bucks at age eighty-five without having put in some investment first.

Consider thinking about your health the same way you think about your finances. Unless you're very young, you've probably already started planning for your retirement and stashing money away. My wife and I met with our financial planner years ago to figure out how much we needed to set aside each month and how to invest it. This makes perfect sense. And it also makes perfect sense to make plans to preserve and protect your health so you can reach age eighty or ninety with a maximum of physical and mental abilities and a minimum of pain. This is particularly important today, as modern medicine has the ability to fix body parts that in past generations might have worn out or shut down. These new techniques can add extra years to your life, but during those additional years the potential for chronic pain can skyrocket. As medicine gets better at prolonging the lives of failing organs, we need to be mindful of how we will live and function with a mixture of strong and not-so-strong "parts."

One of the things that saddens me most is seeing an elderly person who suffers from tremendous discomfort due to the steady deterioration of the body. I ask myself how I can help such a person when the source of the anguish—aging—can't be reversed. I've come to the conclusion that the best way to minimize pain and disability in old age is to take good care of the body throughout life and take special care to prevent the most common sources of age-related chronic pain.

While the potential blessings of being around for an extra decade or two are too numerous to count, the added years also pose new challenges, including how to deal with the pain that might pop up. In chapter 1, I introduced the notion of compressed morbidity. As you recall, James Fries, MD, argued that good lifestyle habits can help you enjoy a very healthy life right until it's time to die. Unfortunately, introducing miraculous medical treatments that preserve worn parts throws a bit of a wrench into the whole compressed morbidity concept.

Must Age = Pain?

The fact of the matter is that growing old is a risk factor for developing chronic pain. The most common "pain culprits" are arthritic joints and a degenerating spinal column. The joints and spine work mighty hard to support the body throughout the eight or nine decades that most people live, but, because of the wear and tear of usage and the strain caused by pushing against gravity to keep the body upright, they also suffer injuries. Just as the soles of your shoes wear out if you wear them long enough, the supporting elements (including the cartilage) in your joints and spine eventually break down. As your natural padding and cushioning give way, things start to grind, get inflamed, and hurt. In addition there are the injuries we all suffer due to trauma. Many of us carry around the scars (inner and outer) of skating crashes, football injuries, motor vehicle accidents, and just plain old falls.

Both of my grandmothers lived well into their nineties, despite being orphans who had very trying life experiences. My maternal grandmother was diagnosed with a problem called *critical aortic stenosis* when she was eighty-three and had to have her aortic valve replaced with a pig valve. Critical aortic stenosis means there is a blockage at the valve that overwhelms the heart's ability to pump enough blood to sustain life.

She was a strong woman who had overcome much in life, so we were not surprised that she lived another ten years—despite a life expectancy of five years tops for the average patient with critical aortic stenosis. This extra ten years blessed all of us with many rewards, including the chance for my own children to know her. Unfortunately, she also had many bad days over those ten years. The arthritis in her knees was so severe that movement was often excruciatingly painful for her. Despite having a grandson who was a well-respected pain doctor, she found there was no magical solution to her problem. The window of opportunity had passed for knee replacements—she was simply too fragile due to her medical condition. There was no compressed morbidity for my grandmother.

I'm afraid situations like this are only becoming more common. Americans over age sixty-five are a large and growing group, and there are an estimated seventy-eight million baby boomers who will keep replenishing the ranks of our senior population for years to come. As medicine gets better and better at prolonging the life of failing organs, we need to begin thinking now—before it is too late—about taking the steps that will allow us to remain healthy, pain free, active, and alert right up until the end of a long life.

Common Sources of Age-Related Pain

The most common sources of age-related pain include problems with the spine, reduced muscle mass, a decline in balance, obesity, arthritis, osteoporosis, and, surprisingly, the mind itself.

Pain Related to the Spine

As we get older the entire spine changes. The protective disks between the vertebrae lose water and thin out, and the cartilage that lines the joints and prevents the bones from rubbing against each other begins to wear away. The net effect is that the spine gets shorter, which causes it to rotate and curve. This is why older people lose height and can become stooped. In effect, their backs are coiling up.

As this process of degeneration and compression takes place, vertebrae can rub together and damage each other. This, in turn, can trigger the growth of bone spurs as the body tries to heal the damaged areas but "grows back" too much bone. Meanwhile, as the spine degenerates it can put pressure on the nerves that are intertwined with the spine, causing neck pain, back pain, or sciatica (back pain with shooting pain down the back of a leg).

None of these structural problems occurs overnight; they develop slowly over a period of many years. As they occur, the rest of the body (including the heart, liver, kidneys, and brain) ages, too. While modern medicine can often keep these organs working well enough to lengthen life, the spine and other tissues continue to wear out, causing chronic pain. So, thanks to medications, an elderly woman with severe spinal deterioration might be able to stay alive for an extra decade. But how will she tolerate living in her body? Too many patients have said to me, "Doc, this ain't living!"

Reduced Muscle Mass and Obesity

As we age, our body composition changes and we naturally lose muscle mass and gain fat. One reason this happens is that the endocrine system changes. The endocrine system consists of the pituitary gland, thyroid gland, pancreas, ovaries, testes, and other glands and tissues that secrete hormones that influence metabolism, hunger, sleep, growth, and sexual development. Women's levels of estrogen and progesterone change dramatically due to menopause, while men experience gradual declines in testosterone levels. These hormonal changes make it harder to maintain muscle mass and, unfortunately, easier to create and store fat around the midsection.

Not only do muscles help us move, they also support the skeleton. The greater the "support load" taken on by the muscles, the less stress the joints have to endure, which helps them last longer. Conversely, as the muscles weaken, the load on the joints increases, ratcheting up the likelihood of arthritis and a decline in the ability of the joints to bear weight. When this happens, it becomes more difficult to participate in weight-bearing activities like standing, walking, running, dancing, and climbing stairs because they become too uncomfortable to tolerate. This can have a devastating impact on your life, for such activities make it possible to buy groceries, visit neighbors, pick up the mail, clean the house, and take care of the garden. As weight-bearing tolerance declines even further, basic activities like getting out of bed, going to the bathroom, and preparing meals can become real struggles. Even in our era of cars, elevators, and motorized scooters, the less you are able to move and walk on your own, the smaller your world becomes. And it can happen surprisingly quickly: Once muscle mass begins to decline, a person can go from shopping at huge malls and hiking in national forests to being confined to home in a relatively short period of time. As the muscles shrink and getting around becomes more and more difficult, you can find yourself interacting with fewer and fewer people and becoming closed off from your community. I've seen far too many people more or less confined to their homes by pain.

A lot of people suffering from chronic pain are above their ideal body weight or are outright obese. Some became heavy before their pain began—and typically gained more once pain became a problem—while others began gaining weight after their pain settled in. In either case I've observed that the longer the pain lasts, the more weight is gained. Of course, the added pounds set these people up for more problems down the line. For example, they may develop back pain that leads to even more inactivity and weight gain, and over the course of ten years that added weight may cause knee pain.

Decline in Balance
As a general rule, balance declines over time. Although this, in itself, is not a cause of pain, it can indirectly bring about pain. Poor bal-

ance is a major factor in limiting your walking tolerance: The more unsteady you feel, the less you'll want to move. And the less you move, the weaker your muscles become and the more likely you are to develop arthritis, obesity, and heart disease. A lack of balance is also a major cause of falls, which in turn are a major source of injury in the elderly. Hip fractures that result from falls are one of the leading causes of hospitalization (three hundred thousand per year) and morbidity in the elderly.

Arthritis

Arthritis is the nation's most common chronic health problem and is the leading cause of disability among those over age fifteen. Technically speaking, the word *arthritis* means "inflammation of a joint," but while some forms of the disease cause a lot of inflammation, others trigger little or none. Broadly speaking, arthritis encompasses some one hundred diseases that attack the joints, from osteoarthritis to rheumatoid arthritis and from gout to ankylosing spondylitis. In its various forms, arthritis afflicts some forty-six million Americans.

Chronic pain, obesity, and arthritis are locked in a vicious circle, with each able to make the others worse. It can go like this: You enter your forties with a little arthritis in your knees, you gain some weight as your metabolism slows, this puts more pressure on your knees and worsens your arthritis, you stop playing racquetball and cut back on your treadmill time because of the pain, now you're burning even fewer calories, so you gain more weight, and so on.

Adding to the misery, in some forms of arthritis—including the most prevalent, osteoarthritis—an additional problem called glycation develops. During glycation, excess glucose circulating in the body binds to certain proteins and fats in the tissues, creating harmful substances called advanced glycation end products, or AGEs. Medical researchers believe that this glycation reaction causes some of the major detrimental changes of aging. Glycation "cross-links" proteins in the body, deforming them and making them less elastic and flexible. On the surface of the body, this cross-linking and deformation shows up as wrinkles. Inside the body, it causes numerous problems including hardening of the arteries, degeneration of the central nervous system, inflammation, and stiff joints. The joints become stiff because the cartilage, which cushions and protects the ends of bones, is made up of collagen, which is susceptible to glycation. In theory, the more sugar that binds to the proteins in the collagen, the stiffer the cartilage will get, and therefore the more painful it will be to move the joint.

Periods of elevated blood sugar increase the rate of cartilage glycation, so it's important to keep blood sugar levels under control. You can use the glycemic index when planning meals to help you select your foods properly and avoid the harmful blood sugar spikes that encourage glycation (see chapter 15 for more information about the glycemic index).

Osteoporosis

Ten million Americans suffer from osteoporosis, and an additional thirty-four million are at greater risk of developing this disease that makes the bones fragile and increasingly likely to break.[19] The disease process itself is painless; you often don't know anything is wrong until a bone breaks. This doesn't mean that all broken bones are the result of osteoporosis, but if you have the disease, your bones will break too easily. For example, if you have osteoporosis, a minor fall that would normally result in nothing more than a bruise might cause your hip to break.

Osteoporosis can affect any bone, but the most serious problems typically occur in the hips or spine. A broken hip can cause prolonged or permanent disability, with the patient confined to a wheelchair, while fractured vertebrae can cause spinal deformity and severe, long-lasting pain.

---

19 National Osteoporosis Foundation. "Fast Facts on Osteoporosis," Accessible at www.nof.org/osteoporosis/diseasefacts.htm. Viewed January 26, 2009.

The disease can strike both sexes, although women are four times more likely than men to develop it. Risk factors that increase the odds of developing osteoporosis include the following:

- Gender (being female)
- Age (being older)
- Ethnicity (Caucasian, Asian, or Hispanic/Latino are at greater risk than African Americans)
- Certain diseases (including anorexia nervosa and rheumatoid arthritis)
- Body type (being small and thin)
- Family history (relatives with osteoporosis or a tendency toward broken bones)
- Personal history (a tendency to break bones, history of skipping periods for women)
- Sex hormone levels (postmenopausal or low estrogen for women, low testosterone and elevated estrogen for men)
- Diet (inadequate intake of calcium and vitamin D, excessive intake of sodium, caffeine, and protein)
- A sedentary lifestyle
- Smoking
- Drinking excessive amounts of alcohol
- Using certain medications (including steroid medications and certain anticonvulsants)

There's nothing you can do about some of these risk factors—you can't change your gender, age, ethnicity, or family history—but you can watch what you eat and make sure that you exercise, two of the best and easiest ways to prevent the disease. A good diet will provide the calcium, vitamin D, vitamin K, and other nutrients needed for strong bones, while regularly engaging in weight-bearing exercise will "stress" the bones and signal the body to keep them strong. It's also a good idea to avoid excessive alcohol intake and smoking altogether. (See chapters 15 and 16 for more about diet and exercise.)

Your Anti-Aging Plan

Change is an integral part of preparing for your pain-free future: Changing your exercise regimen, diet, and/or attitude can put you on the road to good health for years to come. Each individual change does not have to be huge: You don't have to go from being a diehard meat-and-potatoes eater to a strict vegetarian or from an occasional stroller to a marathon runner. You only need a series of small changes to get started—and as you progress, you may find that you enjoy the results of your small changes and want to push them further.

The key elements of an anti-aging plan include proper nutrition and exercise; maintaining a healthy balance between muscle and fat mass; staying ambulatory with good balance; and keeping the mind sharp by stimulating it and keeping it clean with meditative exercises. Naturally you need to develop a strategy that speaks to your biggest needs, yet is doable enough to stay with for years to come.

Walking Tall

I have found the ability to stay ambulatory to be one of the keys to staying young. Over and over again, I've noticed that those who retain the ability to walk have much better "golden" years than those who do not. That's why I consider the ability to walk to be a defining characteristic of graceful aging. Think about it: Standing and walking are necessary for buying groceries, visiting the neighbors, picking up the mail, cleaning the house, and tending the garden. As you go through your fifties, sixties, seventies, and beyond, maintaining your ability to "walk tall," as I say to my patients, means being able to do all of these things. Remember: The less you are able to move and walk on your own, the smaller and smaller your world becomes and the less exercise you can tolerate. Vigorous exercise helps maintain the health of the heart, brain, and just about any other body part that relies on good circulation, so reduced exercise tolerance negatively affects physical and emotional health.

As these changes occur, we interact with far fewer people and become closed off from our communities, which creates a real sense of loss. Even my ailing grandmother, with all of her aches and pains, used to look forward to daily outings with my mom to the local bakery for coffee and human contact. In fact, my other grandmother was famous for keeping her purse and coat next to the front door so she would be ready to leave in an instant with anyone who might be going somewhere. That's why I believe that developing a plan to maintain as much weight-bearing capacity as possible, for as long as possible, should be on the top of anyone's "How to Age Gracefully" list.

The first step toward maintaining the ability to walk tall is to consider how far or how long you'd like to be able to walk. One mile? For thirty minutes? For as long as possible? Are stairs and inclines important to you? The next step is to determine how much you can walk at present. If you are starting off below your target, you have some work to do. If not, if you can already meet your target, then you need to think more in terms of staying fit as you grow older. I say that because preserving your walking tolerance means more than just walking for exercise; it also requires focusing on other important aspects of this chapter, like keeping your joints flexible, balance intact, and muscles strong. Remember: Being a proficient walker when you are *elderly* can make the difference between this being a very rich and fulfilling period in your life or one marked by isolation and lost independence.

Other forms of exercise indirectly contribute to the maintenance of our walking tolerance. For those of us who don't perform hard labor on a regular basis, a consistent strength-training routine is necessary. It's essential that we maintain the strength of our large muscles, like the pectoralis major and minor in the chest, quadriceps and hamstrings in the legs, as well as small muscles like the short fibers between the vertebrae in the spine and the small muscles in the hands. Keeping all your muscles strong greatly increases your chances of feeling good and being ambulatory at a time when your peers might be struggling just to get out of bed.

The exercise plan outlined in chapter 16 is designed to develop overall body strength. Free weights, machine weights, bands, and old-fashioned push-ups and pull-ups are all good strength-training exercises. And just thirty to sixty minutes of this type of exercise twice a week may be enough to prevent age-related decline in the large muscle groups. Focusing on large muscle groups alone, however, ignores the many other valuable muscles necessary for a strong, flexible, and active body. For example, there are dozens of small supporting muscles up and down the spine or in the hands and arms that are not engaged if you focus solely on weight training. These muscles also need to be strengthened and exercised if they are to help the body remain functional.

Yoga and Pilates exercises can help with this. Consider *Downward Dog,* the basic yoga shown in chapter 17. Starting with the hands and moving down to the feet, it is amazing how many muscle groups get engaged in this posture. First of all, the fingers and hands are very active on the floor, which strengthens small muscles in the fingers, hands, and forearms that would likely never get used when lifting heavy weights. The complex muscle groups around the shoulders are active in helping roll the shoulder blades down the sides. As the spine is stretched, numerous muscles up and down the back help support this elongation. Next the pelvis, with its many layers of muscles, has to work to stay elevated. Below the pelvis, the hamstrings work to straighten the legs and support the body weight. Even the small muscles in the feet are activated for support and balance. This simple pose utilizes parts of the body that may be missed with exercises that just focus on specific large muscle groups.

In addition to buffing up the muscles, strength-training exercises also help prevent bone loss and osteoporosis by putting stress on the bones, which encourages the body to strengthen them in response. Of course, the only way that exercise will pay off down the line is if you do it consistently over the course of many years. And that means you'll need to find forms of exercise that are diverse, interesting, and most of all fun! There are all kinds of ways to exer-

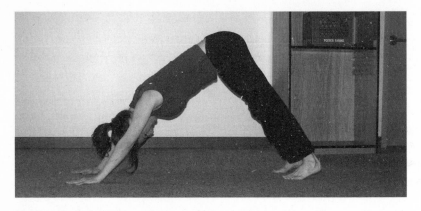

cise, so don't limit yourself. Keep looking for ways to move your body that will be enjoyable—you'll be much more likely to stick with an exercise program that gives you pleasure!

Maintaining and Improving Balance

Balance generally gets shakier with age, but there are plenty of things you can do to maintain and even improve it. Some examples include dancing, riding a bicycle, practicing yoga or tai chi, and doing Pilates (which improves core strength and increases trunk stability).

Simply walking or using exercise machines may not do the trick. To improve your balance you need to perform activities that require your nervous system to "practice" the many minute adjustments it has to make to keep you steady and force you to strengthen the muscles that keep your body stable as you perform various activities. Research suggests that exercise classes that offer a variety of movements will help reduce falls best, so it's a good idea to take a class!

Don't take poor balance lying down! There are simple balance-building exercises you can do at home to get started. For example,

- Stand on one leg for thirty seconds at a time.
- Put your shoes on while standing up.
- Sit down in a chair and get up again, without using your hands for either movement.

- Practice heel-to-toe walking. With each step, land first on your heel then gently "rock" the foot forward until your weight is on the toe. You can put one hand on the wall as you walk to steady yourself, or if need be someone can walk beside you to help keep you steady.
- Do leg lifts with the help of a chair. Stand tall holding onto the back of a secure chair. Raise one knee toward your chest, hold it there for a few seconds, then lower it. Now do the other knee. You can also raise each leg out to the side (without bending the knees), or raise your straightened legs behind you, one at a time, while still holding on to the chair. See if you can build up so that with each leg you are doing each of the three leg lifts ten times each.

Nutrition and Weight Management

Following the principles of the anti-inflammatory diet discussed in chapter 15 will serve you well in your journey toward painless aging. Avoiding spikes in blood sugar by choosing smaller but more frequent low-glycemic meals will reduce the amount of extra glucose floating in the blood. That means there will not be as much glucose to bind to cartilage through the process of glycation. Remember: Aging experts believe glycation is a major contributor to painful, degenerated joints.

As I pointed out at the beginning of this chapter, obesity causes pain directly by stressing the joints and indirectly by increasing the odds of developing a variety of other diseases that lead to pain. Obesity can also make it more difficult for you to move your body, which is another problem. I can't say it enough: Staying healthy as you age depends a lot on maintaining a healthy weight and body mass index.

The anti-inflammatory diet helps prevent weight-related stress on the body by shifting caloric intake away from foods containing trans fats and high fructose corn syrup and toward rainbow foods that are plentiful in antioxidants and fiber. This shift invariably lowers total daily caloric intake, which is a must to counteract the metabolic slowing associated with aging. The abundance of antioxidants serves to clean up toxic waste that can build up in crucial tissues like the heart and brain. A steady flow of proteins during the day keeps important muscle groups fortified.

Although books, newspaper and magazine advertisements, television commercials, infomercials, and your friends may promote this or that fad diet, the truth is this: The best way to lose weight is to burn more calories than you consume. I know it's not very exciting, but this means consuming fewer calories and increasing your energy output. As you age, your metabolism will naturally slow down, which means your body will burn fewer calories than when you were younger. Cutting out just one can of soda or one energy drink each day can reduce your daily caloric intake by 150 calories or more, while walking an additional 30 minutes can burn about 100 calories. That adds up to 250 fewer calories per day. Approximately 3,500 calories equals 1 pound, so at that rate you'll lose 1 pound every 2 weeks.

Of course fad diets promise dramatic weight loss in a much shorter period. Unfortunately, while you may be able to lose a lot of weight quickly on a fad diet, studies show that chances are excellent that you'll gain back all of the weight, plus a little more, within a year or so. The scientific truth is that most fad diets don't work, and those that do only work for a brief period. Once you start eating "normally" again, you'll regain the weight. Sensible, safe, and sound dieting, combined with moderate yet steady exercise, is the *only* weight control prescription that has stood the test of time.

Exercise Your Brain

An important part of aging gracefully involves preserving your mental faculties. I believe that chronic pain is a risk factor for declining cognitive function later in life. Why? Because the physiology of the stress response triggered by chronic pain has been shown to reduce brain function. For one thing, the chronic inflammation associated with stress and chronic pain is now known to be a major contributor to Alzheimer's disease and other forms of dementia. In addition, chronic pain may encourage lifestyle habits that can increase the likelihood of developing dementia or Alzheimer's disease. These include challenging our brains less often than we should, overmedicating, consuming a diet high in free radicals and oxidants, and engaging in too little aerobic activity.

It isn't enough just to pay attention to the parts below the neck. Our brains and bodies need constant tune-ups so they will run smoothly in our later years. Fortunately, there are things we can do every day that can contribute to good cognitive function today and down the line. These include the following:

- Follow an anti-inflammatory diet, like the one described in chapter 15. Let nature's powerful antioxidants quell the damaging inflammatory mediators in your brain and body.
- Engage in some form of vigorous exercise at least twice a week—walking counts! Aerobic activities such as walking and running stimulate the growth of new nervous system cells.
- Exercise your brain by keeping it active. Spend more time reading, writing letters, going to museums and lectures, solving crossword puzzles and Sudoku, and playing games like chess and bridge and less time engaging in more passive pursuits like watching television, mindless Internet surfing, and other couch potato–type activities.
- Keep learning. Never stop challenging your mind. Expose it to new things, like a new language or a new musical instrument. Don't settle for the same television shows, Web sites, or newspapers over and over again. Make time to visit stimulating places and events like museums, concert halls, libraries, lectures, and discussion groups. It's never too late to begin learning!
- Love your neighbor. Thoughts and feelings of affection have been shown to promote the growth of new nervous system cells. I know it sounds corny, but embracing this philosophy leads to many happy returns, including a healthier mind.
- Clear the mind of excessive chatter through regular mindful practices such as meditation, prayer, or yoga.

Take stock of how you use your time each day. Are you performing activities that can stimulate your brain? If not, come up with alternative things to do to boost your brainpower.

Losing cognitive ability rapidly ages you. Even in its early stages, even with just a little memory loss, people feel embarrassed and begin to detach from their friends and family. Increasingly isolated, they can easily become depressed and anxious and lose interest in maintaining their health and in life in general as they withdraw into themselves. In other words, just a little loss of brainpower can set in motion events that can make you feel a lot older than your years and drain enjoyment from your life.

Prevention is the best antidote to dementia that we have. Help ward it off by following the tips above and be sure to socialize with happy, healthy people who are fun to be with. Social contacts matter! A recent study conducted by Harvard and University of California, San Diego, found that happy people tend to hang around with other happy people, so happiness is apparently contagious. However, habits or conditions like smoking and obesity can also be contagious, so choose your companions wisely. Spend as much time as possible with happy, healthy people.

Stick to the Basics

It seems like we've covered a lot, but aging as painlessly as possible boils down to just a few basic principles:

- Adhere to the anti-inflammatory diet.
- Exercise muscles big and small to stay ambulatory.
- Keep your weight under control (shoot for a body mass index within the normal range).
- Maintain your balance.
- Give your brain plenty of exercise.
- Spend time with other happy, healthy people.

These six steps can all work together for your benefit. For example, if you consume a health-enhancing diet and exercise, you're already working to keep your weight under control. And by taking an exercise class with a friend, you can remain strong and engage with others.

I urge you to mold this into your own personalized anti-aging plan; create a health portfolio that will serve you well for a lifetime. As you master each element of your plan, you'll be surprised at how easy it is to do the next one.

You owe it to yourself to remain young and healthy, right up until you've reached a very old age. There are many things in this world that age well, including wine, cheese, and violins. Why shouldn't you be one of them, too?

Excellent Anti-Aging Activities

Activities such as yoga, Pilates, tai chi, and qigong may be the perfect antidote to the aches and pains of getting older. They can help you age gracefully because they help you

- Exercise many muscles, including some that might otherwise be overlooked.
- Improve muscular support to the spine and the joints.
- Improve posture and balance.
- Improve flexibility and prevent painful stiffness that might otherwise limit activity.
- Improve core muscle strength and stability around the midsection, warding off low back pain.
- Release stress and increase relaxation.
- Promote good circulation throughout the body.
- Stimulate the release of endorphins, the body's natural painkiller.
- Prevent osteoporosis.

The anti-aging activities in this chapter will go a long way toward helping you ward off the ill effects of aging and help you avoid the chronic pain that can occur as you mature.

Final Words

Chronic pain has become one of modern society's great tormentors. It often comes with a fast pass ticket straight to suffering and devastation, bringing life as you have known it to a screeching halt. What differentiates chronic pain from other health problems is that it is more than a disease, an injury, or a state of mind; it transcends all of that. Underneath it all, chronic pain is an experience that encompasses many parts of the whole, including physical body, emotions, and thoughts. It touches just about every aspect of life that you can imagine.

Not only is chronic pain a unique and uniquely complex problem, it is also widespread. Statistics suggest that it will afflict one person in every family.

Finding a solution to this devilish situation often proves difficult. I have personally stood on the front lines of the "pain battles" with many patients, watching or helping as they ran a gamut of medication trials, therapies, and procedures. I know how chronic pain can defy attempts to control it, even with the best of intentions and the latest technology. I have come to realize that you can't always eliminate such a complex experience by cutting something out or overwhelming it with chemicals. No, the road to recovery and healing is often more of a process than a special treatment given at a specific point in time.

The good news is that having great health is still within reach. In fact, adopting the lifestyle habits I have described in this book can wash away a good deal of the physical and emotional pain in your life. Take advantage of these lessons, strategies, and steps so that you can regain control of your life. Let your mind help your body heal and vice versa; the connection between the two runs deep. And don't slight "old" approaches like yoga and meditation: The results of new and cutting-edge scientific research are supporting the ideas behind many ancient healing practices and emphasizing that the power for positive change lies within you.

Look beyond the labels others give you, or the fears you harbor inside. See what is possible. Your journey starts with a lone step but will require many more, all built on patience and faith.

Resources

Books

Fincher, Susanne F. *Creating Mandalas*. Boston, MA: Shambhala, 1991.

Ganim, Barbara *Art and Healing: Using Expressive Art to Heal Your Body, Mind and Spirit*. New York, NY: Three Rivers Press, 1999.

Glass, Lee E., Ed. American College of Occupational and Environmental Medicine Practice Guidelines. Beverly Farms, MA: OEM Press, 2004.

Kabat-Zinn, Jon. *Full Catastrophe Living: Using the Wisdom of Your Body and Mind to Face Stress, Pain and Illness*. New York, NY: Delta, 1990.

Makin, Susan R. *Therapeutic Art Directives and Resources*. London, England: Jessscia Kingsley Publishers, 2000.

Malchiodi, Cathy A. *The Art Therapy Sourcebook*. New York, NY: McGraw-Hill, 2006.

Pilates, Joseph and William J. Miller. *Pilates' Return to Life Through Contrology and Your Health*. Presentation Dynamics, 1998.

Saplosky, Robert. *Why Zebras Don't Get Ulcers: An Updated Guide to Stress, Stress Related Diseases, and Coping*. New York, NY: Holt Paperbacks, 2004.

Weil, Andrew. *Healthy Aging: A Lifelong Guide to Your Well-Being*. New York, NY: Anchor Books, 2006.

You can also find a number of CDs, DVDs, and videos on qigong, meditation, and related items at the Exercise to Heal Web site, www .exercisetoheal.com/. These excellent materials were prepared by Lee Holden, an internationally known instructor in meditation, tai chi, and qigong who has appeared regularly on American Public Television and over 105 PBS stations throughout the United States and Canada.

Multidisciplinary Pain Programs
Bay Area Pain & Wellness Center
The center "offers a full complement of pain therapies, from highly specialized interventional treatment, to the most sophisticated inter-disciplinary pathways and programs, to tackling the most complex and challenging pain problems in our society."
15047 Los Gatos Boulevard, #200
Los Gatos, CA 95032
(408) 364-6799
www.bapwc.com/

Johns Hopkins Blaustein Pain Treatment Center
The center's "team of pain medicine specialists provides some of the world's most advanced treatment options in a supportive, compas-sionate environment."
Johns Hopkins Outpatient Center
601 North Caroline Street, Suite 3062
Baltimore, MD 21287
(410) 955-7246
www.hopkinsmedicine.org/pain/blaustein_pain_center/

Mass General Center for Pain Medicine
This center strives "to assemble an individualized and comprehensive plan for optimal pain treatment that will allow each person to return to an optimal level of function in his or her work and personal life."
Massachusetts General Hospital
Center for Pain Medicine

Wang Ambulatory Care Center, Suite 340
15 Parkman Street
Boston, MA 02114
(617) 726-8810
www2.massgeneral.org/anesthesia/index.aspx?page=clinical_
services_pain&subpage=pain

Mayo Clinic's Division of Pain Medicine
The well-known hospital offers a "multidisciplinary, team-based approach to the prevention, evaluation, diagnosis, treatment, and rehabilitation of painful disorders."
Mayo Clinic
200 First Street SW
Rochester, MN 55905
(507) 284-2511
www.mayoclinic.org/anesthesiology-rst/painmed.html

Pain Management Department of the Cleveland Clinic
The clinic assembles "the appropriate interdisciplinary team of healthcare professionals who can best help patients."
For information about clinical locations, call (800) 223-2273, ext. 57370
http://my.clevelandclinic.org/anesthesia/pain_management/default.aspx

Productive Rehabilitation Institute of Dallas for Ergonomics (PRIDE)
PRIDE offers an "inter-/multi-disciplinary team approach to functional restoration" to help those with spinal dysfunction and other musculoskeletal disorders.
5701 Maple Avenue, Suite 100
Dallas, TX 75235
(214) 351-6600
www.pridedallas.com

The Rosomoff Comprehensive Pain Center

A multidisciplinary team of specialists is used to "restore patients to their optimum levels of function, reduce or eliminate pain, reduce or eliminate addictive pain medications, enable patients to become independent of the healthcare system, [and] improve quality of life."
The Rosomoff Comprehensive Pain Center
at the Miami Jewish Home & Hospital at Douglas Gardens
5200 NE Second Avenue
Miami, FL 33137
(305) 532-PAIN (7246)
www.rosomoffpaincenter.com/

Southern California Pain and Wellness Center

A comprehensive treatment center modeled after the Bay Area Pain and Wellness Center.
3444 Kearny Villa Road, Suite 302
San Diego, CA 92123
(858) 874-0033
www.scpwc.com

Pain Associations
American Chronic Pain Association

The association's mission is "to facilitate peer support and education for individuals with chronic pain and their families so that these individuals may live more fully in spite of their pain."
PO Box 850, Rocklin, CA 95677
(800) 533-3231
www.theacpa.org

American Pain Society

The society "is a multidisciplinary community that brings together a diverse group of scientists, clinicians and other professionals to increase the knowledge of pain and transform public policy and clinical practice to reduce pain-related suffering."

4700 W. Lake Avenue
Glenview, IL 60025
(847) 375-4715
www.ampainsoc.org/

International Association for the Study of Pain
This worldwide organization "brings together scientists, clinicians, health care providers, and policy makers to stimulate and support the study of pain and to translate that knowledge into improved pain relief worldwide."
www.iasp-pain.org//AM/Template.cfm?Section=Home

Art Therapy Associations
American Art Therapy Association
The AATA "is an organization of professionals dedicated to the belief that the creative process involved in art making is healing and life enhancing."
11160-C1 South Lakes Drive, Suite 813
Reston, VA 20191
(888) 290-0878
www.arttherapy.org

National Coalition of Creative Arts Therapies Associations
This is "an alliance of professional associations dedicated to the advancement of the arts as therapeutic modalities."
www.nccata.org

Information on Buprenorphine Anti-Addiction Treatment
CRC Health Group
20400 Stevens Creek Boulevard, Sixth Floor
Cupertino, CA 95014
(866) 549-5034
www.crchealth.com/index.asp

Urschel Recovery Science Institute
5939 Harry Hines Blvd, Dallas, TX 75235
(214) 905-5090
www.recovery-science.com/

Acknowledgments

I would like to give my heartfelt thanks and appreciation to my incredible team at the Bay Area Pain and Wellness Center. In particular I would like to recognize my practice partner, John Massey, MD, for his moving contributions to the lives he has touched. Special thanks to Rachel Feinberg, Mai Huong Ho-Tran, Greg Garavanian, Christine Hirabayashi, Karlee Holden-Bianco, Shaylin Ebert, and Scott Abke for their important contributions, insights, and positive energy given to this book.

I would also like to thank Sean Mackey, MD, and David Clark, MD, from the Stanford School of Medicine for sharing their valuable perspectives on their important research; Bill George and Kimberly LeTourneau for their business support and marketing help; Randal Flores and David Sullivan for being willing to share for the good of others; Barry Fox for his editing assistance; and James Hummel for his wonderful illustrations.

Lastly I would like to acknowledge the passion shared for this project by Lara Asher and the team at Globe Pequot Press and my dedicated agent, Andrea Hurst. I am eternally grateful for the faith they have bestowed upon this book as a vehicle to improve the lives of so many who deal with pain on a daily basis.

Index

sleep
> disruptions, 241–43
> falling back to, 246–47
> importance of, 240–41
> tips for better, 243–46

smoking, 31
sodium nitrite, 173
soft drinks, 180
Southern California Pain and Wellness
> Center, 281

spices, 173
spinal fusion, 234
spinal stenosis, 233–34
spine surgery, 46–48, 233–34
spirituality
> benefits of, 97–98
> brain imaging and, 98–99

Stanford Pain Clinic, 91–92
stress
> brain and, 81–82
> dangers of, 79
> definition, 75
> fight-or-flight response to, 75–77
> fitness and, 83–84
> health risks of, 12
> inflammation and, 80–82
> neurogensis and, 87
> oxidative, 83
> physiology of, 77–79
> *Why Zebras Don't Get Ulcers,*
>   74–75

supplements, 184–85
surgery
> chronic pelvic pain, 235
> herniated disk, 233
> hip and knee replacement, 234–35
> questions about, 232–33
> spinal fusion, 234
> spinal stenosis, 233–34
> trigeminal neuralgia, 235

sympathetic nervous system, 78–79

T
tai chi, 209–10, 211–16

Topamax, 44, 45
treatment
> balance and, 129
> benefits of interdisciplinary pain
>   programs, 69–70
> chronic pain programs and, 66–67
> complications and side effects
>   of, 21
> control self assessment, 70
> controlling what is ingested, 129
> correct, 9
> creating healing mind, 127–28
> diagnosis vs. cause, 24–27
> doing something vs. doing nothing,
>   21–22, 27
> eliminating unneeded, 9–10
> failed back syndrome, 48–49,
>   57–58
> gaining perspective and, 130–31
> interdisciplinary pain programs,
>   65–66, 67–70, 279–81
> medical manufacturing profits,
>   46–48
> modifying environment, 130
> nonsurgical, 49–50
> patient education, 13
> physician questions prior to,
>   34–35, 50
> quick fixes, 22–24
> shedding patient role and, 14–15
> social connections and, 128–29
> training for success and, 125–27
> using breath and, 127
> *See also* acceptance; art therapy;
>   breathing; Eastern medicine;
>   evidence-based management;
>   exercise; medication; nutrition;
>   pain management; Western
>   medicine

trigeminal neuralgia, 235
turmeric, 173

V
vegetables, 171–73

About the Author

Peter Abaci, MD, is board certified in anesthesia and pain management by the American Board of Anesthesiology. He has been in private practice since 1996 and is the medical director and cofounder of the nationally recognized Bay Area Pain and Wellness Center, located in Los Gatos, California, where he resides with his wife and two children. Abaci has helped create numerous comprehensive programs to help patients overcome their struggles with chronic pain and improve their well-being, including the acclaimed Functional Restoration Program, and he designed and built a state-of-the-art healing center in 2005. He also serves as a volunteer clinical instructor for the Stanford Pain Clinic.